Quarterly Essay

CONTENTS

Quarterly Essay is published four times a year by Black Inc., an imprint of Schwartz Publishing Pty Ltd
Publisher: Morry Schwartz

ISBN 186 395 3817
ISSN 1832-0953

Subscriptions (4 issues): $49 a year within Australia incl. GST (Institutional subs. $59). Outside Australia $79. Payment may be made by Mastercard, Visa or Bankcard, or by cheque made out to Schwartz Publishing. Payment includes postage and handling.

To subscribe, fill out and post the subscription form on the last page of this essay, or subscribe online at:

www.quarterlyessay.com

Correspondence and subscriptions should be addressed to the Editor at:

Black Inc.
Level 5, 289 Flinders Lane
Melbourne VIC 3000 Australia
Phone: 61 3 9654 2000
Fax: 61 3 9654 2290
Email: quarterlyessay@blackincbooks.com
http://www.quarterlyessay.com

Editor: Chris Feik
Management: Sophy Williams
Production Co-ordinator: Caitlin Yates
Publicity: Meredith Kelly
Design: Guy Mirabella

Gail Bell

One sunny afternoon a week before Christmas I met a gifted young woman at a neighbourhood party. Her thoughts and feelings were lavishly on display, flashing like the sunlight on the sea below, sometimes blinding, sometimes obscured by the tumble of associations welling up around her theme. She was visiting relatives and would return to Sydney the following day.

I observed her over a few hours and we talked for a time. By early evening she had squandered her ration of happiness and was more than a little drunk.

It was impossible not to notice the healed scars on her arms, or to miss her references to Sylvia Plath, suicide and Zoloft.

As the party wound down, she claimed the seat beside me. She'd been listening at a distance when I answered a few questions about work I'd done in drug education. I guessed that she wanted to ask me something personal, about medication. I imagined her overwrought state to be concern over mixing dubious chemicals with the prescribed kind, the quandary many of us find ourselves in. I had no idea she'd already stormed that barricade.

During my leave-taking she stayed close, saying something about wanting to stretch her legs. We walked slowly along the cliff road together and she told me stories about her life, love affairs, elations and frustrations ("the usual mixed bag of angsty 22-year-old stuff and then some"), all the while crying unselfconsciously and wiping her nose and eyes with her forearms.

Not wanting to turn her loose I invited her into my house, found a box of tissues, and listened. Should she stay a slave to a drug like Zoloft because she got a bit messy now and again? What did I think? Her friends who, like her, grew up with the 1994 memoir *Prozac Nation*, were "quite divided on medication". Some disdained antidepressants "partly because of the zombifying effect" or because "they're now seen as a bit tacky or clichéd"; other friends – who were scared by her self-harming – "seemed reluctant to argue against the drug" because they could see she needed help.

"It's the postmodern girl's dilemma," she concluded. "We all know the drugs fuck with your brain, but you need them to get on with your life."

Angie, as I will call her, had just won a fellowship to study overseas, an opportunity she saw as a meaningful turning point. Grasping at the symbolism of renunciation, she wanted to clean her slate of old ways, including medicating her sorrows. She sought a quick answer and I gave one. I advised her against stopping the drug. It was the same advice I might give in the clinical setting of my professional life; *follow the prescription, but if in doubt, go back to your doctor,* the tame dove answers of my white-coat training.

What follows is the longer, vastly more digressive version of a reply I've been formulating for this young woman since she flew off to New York and fell in love with a skyline.

Do I really need the drugs that were prescribed for me? Do I have the right to question medical authority? Am I paying a long-term price for short-term peace of mind? The questions are valid and increasingly common. Our intellect, which likes to assert itself when faith demands we keep silent and take our medicine, will keep on shaping these questions, even in the face of competent reassurance, even when we are told the drugs will save our lives.

Angie's very individual story, which I will come to later, is one of several million Australian stories which lead to the same punch-line: a prescription for antidepressant tablets. In 2004, twelve million prescriptions for this group of drugs were dispensed through the Pharmaceutical Benefits Scheme (PBS), a figure that contains both newly initiated scripts and monthly repeats of established regimes and equates to well over a million annual users. More people than ever before in the history of Australia are taking antidepressants. Five million PBS scripts in 1990, 8.2 million in 1998, twelve million last year, 250,000 of which were written for patients under twenty years old.

It is not surprising within one's own circle to discover that your postman, your bank manager, your best friend, three of your nieces, the surly boy in the next street and even the cat you offer to "sit" while your colleague is away are all on SSRIs. Selective serotonin reuptake inhibitors. Or the newer SNRIs, or NaSSAs. The acronyms matter little beyond the borders of medical jurisdiction. We take the drugs on faith, reassured by the certainties of hard science that seem to beep like text messages from their chemical aliases.

Collectively, these drugs are called psychoanaleptics. They restore, amplify, even (it is claimed) invigorate our impoverished supplies of happy-making brain chemicals. Worldwide, antidepressant sales recently topped twenty billion US dollars annually. From anybody's perspective, this is an impressive expression of faith.

At a time when more and more of our citizens are drawn to the narrowband evangelical message of a personal god who watches over our wellbeing if we dose up regularly on the approved scripture, it is tempting to conceive of mood-altering drugs as secular fetishes for unhappy souls. Except that the potential for harm from prescribed drug-taking is demonstrably higher than it is from handclapping and shut-eye singing in a Pentecostal church.

After a ten-year love affair with "happy pills", we are beginning to see flaws in some of the hard science underpinning our beliefs about the safety of these drugs, and to recognise the disguised motives of those who bring the drugs to market. Researchers are questioning the wisdom of medicating 10 per cent of the population with potent molecules when (many argue) other, less encroaching strategies might work just as well. Doubt is not a comfortable place for the growing membership of the second-wave Prozac nation, who are beginning to wonder whether they've jumped aboard a bandwagon for no good purpose.

The counter view to this concern, championed and buttressed by most physicians and all drug companies, is an appeal to our collective sense of perspective: the increase should not be couched in terms of over-prescribing but as a "catch-up effect" after decades of under-diagnosis and under-prescribing. By 2020, we are told, depression is expected to constitute the biggest burden on health spending in the Western world.

Looking back at the last decade, it now seems as if an epidemic has slipped in under the usual radar screens and multiplied, secretly. Twelve million prescriptions for antidepressants in a population of less than twenty million? If the number of prescriptions truly reflects the numbers who are depressed, then we may need to re-design our tourist brochures. The sun-bronzed Aussie optimist with his no-worries attitude to calami-ty might be an outdated caricature. We may need to position our national larrikin on a bleak promontory, hands deep in his pockets, hood pulled over his head, contemplating a leap into oblivion.

And yet, glancing around the new psychopharmacologised neighbour-hood, it would seem that all was well. The postman is whistling, the bank manager is back at work, the best friend is taking yoga classes, the nieces are crying less and the cat has stopped licking itself into hairlessness.

Overlooked, perhaps forgotten, in the neighbourhood snapshot above is the surly boy in the next street. About him, we should worry. He is eighteen and he is not whistling. His symptoms are so severe, so disabling, so manifestly black that he can't get off his bed. He may have already attempted suicide, he will certainly be hospitalised again in the near future. At the outset of this essay it is important to reserve a front-row seat for the severely depressed patient, drowning, in William Styron's words, under a "toxic and unnameable tide that obliterate[s] any enjoyable response to the living world". This boy is not representative of patients who want to feel "better than well", the Prozac warcry. He is someone who cannot remember what "well" feels like, he is the patient for whom the mood-enhancing drugs were invented, but who (curiously) represents only a small proportion of the millions of users.

Is alarm the correct response to this increase in prescription numbers? If drugs make our citizens happy and functional, what's all the fuss about? Alarm is a response to threat, and like many Australians who have been alerted to perceived threats in recent times, I am curious about this strange beast haunting the neighbourhood.

After many years of working in pharmacies and around pharmacology, it has taken me a few years of reduced involvement (working two days, then one day a week) to notice that on balance I have become the air I breathed in thirty years of dispensing, to acknowledge that a kind of pharmaceutical ectoplasm has stuck to my skin, that allopathic rhetoric has colonised my thinking and left me with an acquired pro-drug bias.

And I am not alone in almost involuntarily associating illness with a drug cure. Many ask if the antidepressant epidemic has been inadvertently conjured up by doctors reaching too quickly for their prescription pads.

Others blame the tactics of the big drug companies who have been selling the message that depression is underdiagnosed. "A lot of money can be made from healthy people who believe they are sick," is the message of Ray Moynihan's comprehensive work on the phenomenon he calls "selling sickness" and author Lynn Payer called "disease mongering". Are commercial pressures and drug company profiteering driving the escalation in prescription numbers? Could the answer be so simple?

Or, is another perspective required? Do we need to turn our gaze back upon ourselves, the patients who knowingly walk into the surgery with a prescription-outcome in mind?

Australians are avid supporters of drug therapies. In 2004 we spent three billion dollars on prescription drugs. Of the top fifty most-prescribed drugs on the Pharmaceutical Benefits Scheme to June 2004, four were antidepressants: citralopam (Cipramil) 16th, sertraline (Zoloft) 25th, paroxetine (Aropax) 27th, venlafaxine (Efexor) 46th. Zoloft was top of the pops for nearly a decade but is coming off patent this year and, like an ageing star, has had to make way for younger, hotter rivals.

In fact, rather than rising and rising, we are witnessing the teetering (some say, about to crash) crest of a wave of SSRI use, a wave that assumed its massive shape and rose skywards from 1990, as antidepressant use increased by 352 per cent over a decade, then levelled out. Market saturation may be a factor in the slowdown (the SSRI market is young relative to the tricyclic boom that came before it). Alternatively, the absence of a new blockbuster like Prozac (1990) or Zoloft (1996) coming onto the stage may account for the plateau. We may just be waiting for the next star to appear.

Social scientists have been keeping an eye on the depression phenomenon for the past decade. Rapid social change is taking its toll. As a nation we're profoundly disturbed by the acceleration of change, the shrugging off of methods and manners that have served us well, the feeling that many of us are somehow failing to meet modern challenges, that we have a new malaise called, by Hugh Mackay, "change fatigue".

The medical profession is well aware of this, but the question is what it thinks it is seeing. The impediments to recognition owe much to the adage about the forest and the trees. A diffuse systemic problem, as physicians know, is often harder to diagnose and treat than a visible affliction.

I want to suggest that this impressive, noticeable increase in antidepressant usage in Australia today has come about through the co-operation of three large but inherently unequal groups: the multinational drug companies; the physicians who write prescriptions; and the public who turn to medicine for answers.

And that driving this closed system (which resembles the hypothesised neural loop that makes us depressed and keeps us there) is uncertainty about the way we are governed, and the impact of world events on our personal resilience.

The epidemic of antidepressant-taking (the phenomenon which alarms us) is analogous to the disease itself. There are gradations, complexities and dimensions to the treatment which must be understood before we look to a solution. We at least have to catch the beast and study its habits before we load up the shotgun.

The history of medicine is an unfolding story of orthodoxies that have been superseded. In 1621, when Robert Burton drew together the threads of all that had been written about melancholy in his magisterial book *The Anatomy of Melancholy*, the condition was thought to be caused by a cold, thick, dry, black, sour fluid called a humour located in the inner brain. Melancholy's outward expression, in the language of Burton, was "fear and sadness without any apparent occasion"; its inward source, "anguish of the mind". I have a great affection for Burton's book, not least because it reminds me that human unhappiness has not altered profoundly over the centuries; that we are not looking at some newly hatched, precocious monster called "depression" that is greedy for our small measure of contentment.

Today's medical expert will confidently describe the anatomy of depression in more stringent language. It is a disorder of mood. It may occur only once in a lifetime, but is more commonly recurrent; it is familial; is related but not tied to personality type; is more common in women; and has many well-known symptoms, the predominant one being the loss of capacity to experience pleasure. It is not a one-size-fits-all condition. There are variants which are given different designations; there are progressions that can occur from the unipolar type (depression only) to the bipolar type (cycling depression and mania). Underlying all of the outward expressions, we are now told (the great breakthrough in understanding), is a deficiency of certain neurotransmitters in the synapses or spaces between nerve endings in the brain. When the balance is out of kilter, we lose our sense of wellbeing.

When I was a student, we used other words to circle around the nebulous idea of depression. *Exogenous*, coming from an external source, like grief, divorce, retrenchment; and *endogenous*, coming from within with no apparent cause. Sadness or "normal" depression was in the '70s (and still is) a universal human response. We went through "holiday blues, anniversary reactions, maternity blues" but these were transient passages, and not considered to be psychopathologic unless they persisted beyond accepted time limits. If they did, you had clinical depression. This was a "morbid state", limited to those individuals with a special vulnerability.

"Guilty rumination and self-reproach are more characteristic of depressions in Anglo-Saxon cultures," my 1970s *Manual of Diagnosis and Therapy* informs me.

Subjectively, depression is a bleak, lonely place haunted by fears of impending tragedy and intimations of going mad.

Burton and others, while acknowledging the depths to which the depressed person may sink, discovered compensations. Melancholy was a "disease of superior wits", and in the more profound cases he often found "the spark of genius". Four centuries later, author Elizabeth Wurtzel was ambivalent about vacating her mansion of depression when offered a new drug, Prozac. She wrote, in *Prozac Nation*:

> In a strange way, I had fallen in love with my depression ... I loved it because I thought it was all I had. I thought depression was the part of my character that made me worthwhile ... the by-products of depression seemed to keep me going. I had developed a persona that could be extremely melodramatic and entertaining. It had, at times, all the selling points of madness, all the aspects of performance art.

An old idea, made current by recent work in evolutionary psychology, suggests that depression may be adaptive, a feature included in the basic physiological package of every human because it has a survival value. The controversial work of Edward Hagen, Paul Watson and Paul Andrews suggests that there are gains from moderate depression (people respond to your cry for help; you buy yourself time to think your way out of problems) and even hereditary benefits from the worst outcome of major depression — suicide — in a harsh and controversial theory which sees suicide as adaptive: "Get rid of yourself and let your relatives get on with gene population."

Paul Watson made the following prediction:

> Within the next 50, 100, 200 years, it doesn't really matter, the pharmaceutical industry is going to have our neurochemistry down to the point where they will be able to save us from having any adverse experience whatsoever, no matter how our life is actually going. Before we start turning off all these unpleasant experiences, we need to know what those unpleasant experiences are for – to understand what the potential function of depression is in human life.

Other scientists (and most physicians) are scathing about this proposition. "If it ever was a survival mechanism, it is now one that should be sloughed off along with full body hair and prehensile toes," comments Rita Carter in her book *Mapping the Mind*.

A backward glance alerts us that medical entrepreneurs have confidently predicted drug-based cures for depression since antiquity, but never with such confidence as the mid-twentieth century, after Freud, when psychotropic drugs began to play a significant part in depression therapy. The dynasty of drugs which began with lithium in 1949 was strengthened a few years later by the first of the tricyclic antidepressants, imipramine (Tofranil); then, in 1955, market control was enlarged and fortified by the introduction of amitriptyline (Tryptanol), which reigned over all competitors for thirty-five years.

The arrival of Prozac in 1990 changed all that. Prozac, the first SSRI, rapidly moved to the top of the popularity lists and engendered multiple copies and improvements on the original. By 2002, there were twenty-one different antidepressants marketed in Australia.

The claims of brain scientists to understand the mysteries of mood are not, and never have been, proven beyond all doubt. But the invisible circuitry of the brain is slowly yielding to neuroscientists using the latest imaging scanners. In predictions which are open to both sinister and auspicious interpretations, brain mappers are painting a new treatment picture in which "an individual's mind (and thus behaviour) will be almost entirely malleable."

When the link between serotonin (and other transmitters) and mood was made, we moved from "mechanism of action unknown" (as it was for the tricyclics) to not only is it known, but *we can target the exact spot*. From this exact targeting we come to the word "selective". Selectivity is a powerful marketing tool. It's an heroic claim by the scientists, taken up by the spinmeisters at the drug company and broadcast in capital letters. Within its bold claim to selective powers are echoes of advertising hype, the notion that newer is better, targeting is better than scatter bombing, that they, the inventors, have found something which supersedes all that has gone before.

For a symptom like high blood pressure, or high cholesterol, the rationale for opting for drug therapy is well understood inside and outside the medical profession. High numbers are bad. A drug that brings the numbers down is good. Even with only the most basic understanding of what a systolic pressure of 190, or a cholesterol reading of 7.2, might mean in physiological terms, the layman needs no further persuasion to stay on his pills than to see the numbers drop before his eyes.

The more difficult, less quantifiable, phenomenon is our sense of wellbeing. There is no screening tool, no radiological marker, no rash or swelling that definitively diagnoses a plummet or disintegration in our sense of ourselves – a condition which has gone by many names but which now washes up in medical lexicon as clinical depression.

Pharmacotherapy alone, without a retinue of adjuncts like cognitive therapies and lifestyle changes, squeezes out any other definition or understanding of what happiness is. It positions us in the area of bio-reductionism. We are our hormones. We are our neurotransmitters. It silences other voices. Happiness, the message seems to say, is only possible as long as the neurotransmitters are flowing.

It is perhaps useful to remember that until the nineteenth century the general community, and micro-communities like the family, dealt with "mad", "bad" and "sad" people. Gaols or religious institutions housed the socially outcast. The profoundly melancholic might have been bled by a physician, or sent to the country for a taste of farm life and fresh air to doctor their sullen ruminations.

Increasingly, emotional dis-ease has migrated from the aegis of traditional healers and listeners into the offices of medical practitioners whose capacity to hear out the complex unfolding of stories of anguish or loss is limited by time constraints and the pressure of a full waiting room.

Making an appointment with your GP may not be the definitive answer to the question *where do I go when I feel depressed?*, but it's the best address on offer at the moment. Most episodes of depression are diagnosed and treated in a primary care facility. Eighty-five per cent of PBS-subsidised prescriptions for antidepressants are written in general practice rooms.

There is an anomaly in this state of affairs. "There is no evidence to support the use of antidepressants in general practice patients who do not meet the criteria for major depression or dysthymia." And yet the type of depression that arrives in a GP's office is rarely "major" in the strict sense of the definition. The patient may be "flat as a piece of paper", "weepy", "sleep-deprived", "lacking in libido" "socially withdrawn", but is not, in the main, the deeply depressed patient seen in secondary and tertiary care facilities. A quick check in the PBS Guidelines shows clearly that SSRIs and the newer drugs are only licensed for major depression and a few variants like obsessive-compulsive disorder (OCD). In fact, Kelsey Hegarty writes in *Australian Prescriber*, "all the testing on the efficacy of antidepressants was done on patients in secondary and tertiary settings who had major depression," and further, "there is no good evidence to support the use of antidepressants in minor depression."

And yet the stratospheric increase in antidepressant prescribing tells us that doctors (and patients) have enthusiastically bought into the message that drugs defeat depression. The loop that begins in scientific research, winds through drug company development and spin, snakes into the doctor's surgery, and lassos the patient in the chair, is pulled outside into the community where it is threaded from hand to hand, as happy patients tell others that a drug has fixed their lives. Few people argue with the results of SSRI drug therapy. It seems to work for mild depression – the sort of normal sadness that afflicts us all, the people with low-level sorrow. Sometimes, a course or two will act as a bridge for someone who cannot find his way out of the mire, and physicians report that they are happy to discontinue the drugs when their patients are stable again.

Digging a little deeper one finds that each transformed patient has paid a small price for mood enhancement – not a large dollar price compared to, say, the United States, but in the form of "start-up" side effects. Each has accommodated up to two weeks of nausea, trouble falling asleep or staying awake, constipation and sometimes its opposite, waning of an already underactive libido and perhaps an increase in anxiety. This spectrum of complaints is marketed to the patient as a kind of endurance test. Are you man or woman enough to put up with a bit of initial discomfort for the ultimate good that awaits you after six to twelve months of daily tablet swallowing? For some, the start-up effects are so awful they prefer to revert to the vague sense of unhappiness that brought them to the doctor in the first place. Feeling "lost and flat" is suddenly preferable to feeling "weird" because of a drug.

In my own questioning of the anomaly I've yet to find an answer that isn't contradictory. Yes, say the prescribing doctors, strictly speaking it is true that we should only use SSRIs for major depression; yes, it's true they're not licensed for minor to moderate depression; yes, we use them for minor to moderate cases; yes, they work, and no, we are not breaking any rules.

The contradiction seems to be semantic: the word "major" has taken on another meaning in the general practice setting. A depression qualifies as major if it has gone on for longer than two weeks, is interfering with the patient's daily life, and is physically manifested by sleeping problems, appetite changes and libido swings.

All those symptoms, I contend, could be ascribed to falling in or out of love, facing end-of-year exams, growing older or getting hung-up on office politics. This is ordinary life angst repackaged in a medical presentation. Giving a patient a potent drug to soothe what are often transient worries is the legacy of listening too attentively to the *lesser* things that commend its use (once-a-day dosage, kind to the stomach, PBS-listed, longer-acting, shorter-acting, faster excretion – all of which are noteworthy and attractive in and of themselves) at the expense of what is essential and absolute about a drug: its need to exist in the first place, and its necessary and proven applicability to a pathological condition.

The lesser things about a drug are details. And we delight in the vocabulary: selective, inhibitory, reversible, stimulant. When a drug company representative calls with a new drug (or an established one that needs bolstering because a competitor has reared its head), the verb used to describe their pitch is "detailing". And while this presentation of favourable aspects helps the medical and paramedical professions to fit the drug into a category (for example, Lexapro the new and better Cipramil), it avoids the larger question: why does the drug exist *per se*? Detailing helps a busy practitioner only in secondary and subsidiary ways; it intrudes lesser things into his or her field of vision, even distorts the perspective, leaving the more important consideration kaleidoscoped through a prism of shiny new information.

In his 1961 book, *The Myth of Mental Illness*, Thomas Szasz identified among his colleagues a binary division in approaches to treating mental disorders. He called one group the organicists, or scientists who believed that mental diseases are disorders of the brain. The second group, which he designated humanists, believed in "the power to explain the observed and to influence it".

Belief in this dichotomy has persisted into the new millennium, with more than just a change of labels. The lines are now drawn between biopsychiatrists and psychoanalysts, between Prozac and Freud, between drug doctors and talk doctors. The division has been financially material to the pharmaceutical industry. In terms of drug company dollars, only the first group – in corporate parlance – is "worth the spend".

Research into brain chemistry had to deliver some good reasons for pharmaceutical companies to get involved in the depression business. There was a time when mood drugs were slow movers off the warehouse shelves. Part of the problem was the vague understanding of what neurotransmitters actually did in the mood cycle.

Here is a story that pre-dates Prozac by forty years, but heralds what was to come when a big drug company got a sniff of the big money. In the 1950s when the first tricyclic, imipramine (Tofranil), had been out there for a while doing modest business for Geigy, Merck was pursuing strategies for marketing its forthcoming tricyclic, amitriptyline (Tryptanol). Depression, in the 1950s, was still seen as a symptom, not a disease, so Merck employed its best lateral thinkers to address the puzzle and come up with a specific selling angle. A drug, like a smart bomb, has to have a target, and the parties concerned (physician and patient) have to believe in the science guiding the drug inexorably towards its bullseye. How do you sell a drug to doctors when they're not sure of its exact role or clinical application? You remove the fuzziness around the definition of depression. You label it as a disease. The reconceptualisation of depression as a disease renders it visible to medicine's gaze.

Merck purchased 50,000 copies of a book called *Recognizing the Depressed Patient* which gave general practitioners a clear guide to diagnosing depression, and distributed the book to GPs along with the usual free drug samples and brochures. Tryptanol took off like a rocket. Thirty years later amitriptyline was still the number one-selling antidepressant in the business. In 1992 it remained hovering at the top, four places above Prozac, the bright new star that would rapidly eclipse its popularity but never eliminate it. Today, amitriptyline still ranks at the lower end of the top ten.

The collective name for the largest pharmaceutical companies is big pharma. The top five corporations to November 2004 were Pfizer, Glaxo-SmithKline (GSK), Merck, AstraZeneca and Novartis. These are very rich, very successful companies that measure their turnover in hundreds of billions of dollars. Globally, antidepressants were the overall number three bestsellers in their top ten earners last year.

Big pharma's top executives and CEOs receive handsome salaries and stock options, as one would expect, and within the gleaming walls of these monoliths labour an army of executives, lawyers, marketing geniuses, salaried scientists, product champions, thought leaders, and public relations experts rarely seen in the public domain, never seen in the GP's office or the pharmacy, and not found within cooee of the end-receiver, the customer.

Drug companies are rich because they excel at what they do. Once upon a time what big pharma did was to discover new drugs, but since 2002 fewer significant new products have been reaching the markets. For drug companies, the fight for market share is changing. It is no longer enough to switch patients from the competitor's brand to theirs; the aim of the game is to increase the size of the market, and the most effective way of doing that is by enlarging the target for their existing drugs. Depression as a single entity is enlarged into subgroups: depression with obsessive-compulsive disorder, school phobia, panic attacks, social phobia, bulimia. The list is growing. It is no secret that drug companies actively court the busy community physician with simplified messages about niche conditions. Variants like obsessive-compulsive and panic disorders, the drug reps say, can be confidently managed by Zoloft or Aropax or Cipramil.

The multinationals have taken the pulse of the worried well (Freud's term) and invested millions of dollars in simplifying a profoundly complex mental condition into a set of keywords and bullet-point brochures, which, like a biological feedback mechanism, provide the professional at the coalface with a ready comeback for his patient. GPs in Australia have grown more confident in prescribing SSRIs because this group of drugs has been sold into surgeries on the back of claims to selectivity. It must be difficult indeed for an overworked GP to forget the drug option when his office is strewn with advertising's best-presentation product reminders.

In 1996 Pfizer Inc., New York, through its then chairman and CEO, announced the company's "clear strategic focus to discover, develop, and bring to market innovative products that address major unmet health care needs". Pfizer was exceedingly happy to record the US Food and Drug Administration's approval of the use of Zoloft for obsessive-compulsive disorder. "Dr Niblack (head of Research & Development, R & D) described the company's strategy for sustained output of innovative therapies. The keys to this strategy, he said, are an emphasis on the early stages of the R & D pipeline, while continually adding extra value to Pfizer products already on the market, for example, the new indication for Zoloft."

Note the phrase "unmet health care needs". This often translates into "yet to be invented needs". Within a few years, the "extra value" Zoloft coefficient increased with an approval for "panic disorder where other treatments have failed or are inappropriate". Over time, the indications for Zoloft broadened to include post-traumatic stress disorder, social anxiety disorder, premenstrual dysphoric disorder and premature ejaculation. The rise and rise of Zoloft almost eclipses its predecessor, Prozac, and so far, Zoloft has not had the bad press that eventually sidelined that drug.

I have been navigating the Pfizer website, noticing its mix of hype, implied benevolence, examples of philanthropy, free advice, cross-promotional endorsements and links. The link to *Silent epidemic of depression associated with arthritis* is a classic example of what is called in pharmacy "companion selling", a tactic that translates into big dollar sales for Pfizer, which markets both Zoloft for depression and Celebrex for arthritis. "National polling by Arthritis Australia and Pfizer Australia links arthritis with depression," the report reads. "Depression is an illness, so if you feel depressed the sooner you seek treatment, the sooner you find relief."

The site has all the charm of any promotional brochure, and is really not worlds away from the websites of other highly successful corporations. Publishing for instance. Or banking. It has success written all over its smooth surface.

In the we-earn-our-profits model that drug companies present, one of their biggest outlay costs is claimed to be in the area of research and development. In 2001, a monetary value of US$802 million was put on the cost of bringing one new drug to the market. In the US, this figure has been used as a powerful justification for the continued high prices of drugs: "Implicit in this claim is a kind of blackmail: If you want drug companies to keep turning out lifesaving drugs, you will gratefully pay whatever they charge." Dr Marcia Angell, former editor-in-chief of *The New England Journal of Medicine*, uncovered deception in these figures, and misrepresentation of the amounts spent on genuine R & D. The top ten US drug companies spent, for instance, 14 per cent on R & D, and more than twice that amount (31 per cent) on marketing and administration. The breakdown of how each company allocates its money is not made available to outsiders (or to most company insiders). These facts are "in a black box, hidden from view", which, as the author points out, is a strange obfuscation given that the high cost of drugs is justified by the company's expenses on research.

A spokesperson for Pfizer Australia, our biggest drug company, told me it was "a nonsense that Pfizer spent more on marketing than R & D.

Have a look at the motor industry. Nobody gets stuck into them." Indeed. Drug companies are not unique in their use of clever tactics to win sales.

But there is a telling point to be made here about penalties. The conduct of drug companies is highly regulated in Australia with screeds of restrictions on what is permissible inside its codes of practice. The *Poisons Act*, the *Trade Practices Act* and the Commonwealth and State *Therapeutic Goods Acts*, as well as the international manufacturers' association code of practice must all be adhered to. Overseeing the statutory requirements is the industry's peak body and chief regulator, Medicines Australia (known until July 2002 as APMA).

Medicines Australia makes some impressive claims for its manufacturing members — they are described as research-based pharmaceutical companies which "discover, develop and manufacture prescription medicines. Medicines [that] save lives, reduce and cure diseases and limit Federal and State Governments' expenditure on [more expensive] treatments such as surgery, hospitalisation and increased aged care."

One is a little surprised to read, in Section 12, *Sanctions*, that the penalties for breaches of its code attract a maximum fine of $200,000 and a recommendation to the Board for possible suspension if warranted. Surprised because the fine is so small when measured against the listed company profits, and the noble life-saving ideals they espouse.

Pharmacists, including myself, see many of the same drug reps who detail doctors. The visits are courtesy calls to alert buyers that a particular drug has been detailed to nearby medical practices (invariably, if the rep has done her job, this results in a temporary increase in scripts), and to drop off literature, enrolment forms, and to ask for the comparative sales figures of their brand and their competitor's. "How is my drug doing?" they will ask, and in the main, we give an answer. Pharmacists receive small tokens (smaller than those given to doctors) like pens, sticky notes, writing pads, calendars (as I type, I am resting the heel of my right hand on an ergonomically pleasing mouse pad provided by my Pfizer rep).

Occasionally, where the relationship is warm, it might also stretch to a sponge cake and lamingtons for morning tea.

In a 1998 study, six influence techniques were identified in encounters involving pharmaceutical reps and medical practitioners. The giving of gifts, for instance, called by the authors the technique of reciprocity, creates a sense of indebtedness in the physician, a debt which realistically can only be honoured by prescribing the company's products. The technique of friendship/liking is "potentially very powerful" and in my own experience, and the experience of GPs I know, probably the strongest incentive to co-operate with requests (e.g. to provide pharmacy computer data on rival brands). The other techniques: commitment/consistency (appealing to our need to be consistent), social validation (conforming to established practices), authority (believing claims attributed to experts without really checking) and scarcity (get in before the supply runs out), may be said to be common across a wide spectrum of commercial businesses that employ reps. Why then is the practice on the nose in the context of pharmaceuticals?

Marcia Angell puts it this way: "If prescription drugs were like ordinary consumer goods, all this might not matter very much. But drugs are different. People depend on them. People need to know that there are checks and balances on this industry so that its quest for profits doesn't push every other consideration aside." Especially, one might argue, for drugs which act inside the delicate skull-bound organ we cannot live without, and would not want tampered with for no good reason.

Pharmaceutical marketing focuses on what is known (and considered marketable) about a new drug; but we are often not told about risks that are known and have been deliberately omitted from the selling message.

Prozac is old news now. At the beginning of its meteoric rise in Australia our early warning systems were detecting a modest 388 reports (comprising 849 adverse reactions) – including suicidal thoughts, and strange bouts of restlessness (akathisia) – which largely went unremarked. The US count is now somewhere of the order of 45,000 adverse reports filed with the Federal Drug Administration (FDA), and some 2,500 deaths are alleged to be Prozac-related. A quick snapshot of the things we weren't told but which are coming to light now through lawsuits in the US reveals the duplicity at work in clinical trials and in the passage from laboratory to published paper.

In 1978 the first human subjects signed up for the pharmaceutical company Lilly's clinical trials of Prozac. The very first person to receive the drug experienced "dystonia resembling an extrapyramidal reaction", which means abnormal sometimes jerking movements resulting from alterations in muscle tone. In fact, mental and physical agitation were commonly reported adverse reactions (and still are today with the newer SSRIs). The worry, of course, is that mental agitation is a possible precursor to suicide. In 1984 Lilly reported to the FDA that benzodiazepines like Valium and other sedatives were being given with Prozac throughout the trials to offset the stimulant effect.

From 1986 Lilly controlled the flow of information to the FDA. Fearing that the company would "go down the tubes", to quote its in-house top scientist, the company's management instructed that the suicide data on Prozac was not to be evaluated. Then in 1990 Lilly added "suicidal ideation" to its post-marketing reports, but downplayed the significance of this with the counterclaim that feeling suicidal and/or hostile was part of the depressed patient's condition, not a drug side effect. The FDA, which was made aware of the suicide link after an epidemiological study, ignored or discounted the dangers. The actual data showed that suicidality in Prozac patients was 3.6 times greater than for patients taking tricyclics. The famous Joseph Wesbecker court case ensued, Eli Lilly & Co. won in the end, but the great Prozac Goliath was wounded and never fully recovered.

If we can't rely on the FDA or Australia's equivalent regulatory body, the Therapeutic Goods Administration, to pass on what it knows about drug company dishonesty to doctors and consumers, the perpetuation of misinformation is guaranteed.

Marcia Angell spells out the dubious tactics employed at the top levels in the US:

> When a drug company applies to the FDA for approval of a new drug, it is required to submit results from every one of the clinical trials it has sponsored. But it is not required to publish them. The FDA may approve the drug on the basis of minimal evidence ... Companies only publish the positive results, not the negative ones. Often they publish the positive results more than once in slightly different forms in different journals. This practice leads doctors to believe that the drugs are better than they are, and the public comes to share this belief on the basis of media reports.

The inflation of good results and the suppression of inconvenient findings has led in some cases to needless suffering, even death, for consumers.

The recent case of rofecoxib (Vioxx) is instructive. Hailed as the new best thing for arthritis, Vioxx was listed on the PBS in 1999. I remember the campaign and the impressive claims made for the drug. One of the slogans was "kind to the stomach", and I personally suggested to patients (including, as it happens, my mother and mother-in-law) who were experiencing stomach pain from their older medications that they discuss Vioxx with their doctor. Here was a COX-2 selective non-steroidal anti-inflammatory drug, with stated lower risks of gastrointestinal toxicity. The uptake was spectacular. Vioxx prescriptions peaked quickly. Two million prescriptions were recorded in the June 2004 annual PBS statistics, making Vioxx the ninth-highest-volume drug, five places behind (and gaining on) Celebrex, its rival.

Then in October 2004 the bad news was delivered: Vioxx increased the risk of heart attack and stroke, and the drug was abruptly withdrawn.

In fact the first intimations of trouble had appeared twelve months after the drug was listed. A study found a significantly higher incidence of myocardial infarction – that is, heart attack – among patients treated with Vioxx 50mg per day than among those taking naproxen (Naprosyn) 1000mg per day. Four times the incidence. But Vioxx remained on the market because it was not clear what the results were due to: an increase in the risk of thrombosis caused by Vioxx, or a protective effect from Naprosyn, or both.

Serious adverse effects can emerge *after* new drugs are on the market. Ten per cent of FDA-approved drugs in the US between 1975 and 1999 had serious safety warnings added after approval to market was given, and 3 per cent were withdrawn from sale.

Between 2000 and 2004, Vioxx was studied using epidemiology and post-marketing surveillance, culminating in a placebo-controlled trial that established the increased risk of heart problems after 18 *months* of taking the drug.

How, we have every reason to ask, could this have happened? Three important factors were identified. The first was the small sample size of people trialled on Vioxx before it was put on sale. The second was the short trial period (less than six months on rofecoxib, and six weeks on placebo). The third, which is as disquieting as the others, was the type of patient selected for the trial, patients who did not reflect the wider population for whom the drug was intended, that is, middle-aged to elderly citizens with arthritis. None of these matters constituted a code violation according to Medicines Australia or the Therapeutic Goods Administration. Marketing drugs too early, testing them on an unrepresentative trial group and using shortened trial periods are far from unusual practices for drug companies. The system allows it, and when things go very wrong, as they did with Vioxx, a collective shudder ripples through the drug company concerned (Merck), the medical world and the duped public, but nothing, it seems, can stop the 800-pound gorilla (as Marcia Angell calls big pharma) doing what it wants to do.

In 2001, pharma sales worldwide grew by 12 per cent. Global anti-depressant sales grew by 20 per cent. "The sustained growth of the world pharmaceutical market shows that healthcare professionals continue to appreciate the value of pharmaceuticals as a convenient cost-effective form of treatment," said the president of Cambridge Pharma Consultancy. The future, he summed up, looked "positive". The greatest challenge big pharma faced was getting a better return on growing marketing and sales expenditure.

The other players in the drug market are the generic companies. Business is good for the two biggest generic firms in Australia, Arrow and Alphapharm.

The strategies for marketing generics are rather different from those for branded, patented drugs. The aim is to do a good deal with a pharmacy which will substitute the generic brand for the original – where substitution is permitted (by the doctor) and desired (by the patient). When Arrow began to market the anti-cholesterol drug Simvar, participating pharmacies received faxes congratulating them on their conversion rates, that is, swapping patients from the "more expensive" brand (Zocor) to a generic. "Your February conversion rate of 83 per cent means you have won! Your prize will be delivered over the coming month by your representative." In a follow-up fax, pharmacists read: "You and your staff have done all the hard work switching your customers to Simvar. Now it's time to focus on a new opportunity: it's called Xydep (sertraline)." Xydep is Arrow's brand of Zoloft, Pfizer's hit antidepressant. In fact it is the same drug, made by Pfizer, just repackaged as a generic.

Prizes from Arrow are rather more substantial than a bunch of pens. *Competition: what do you think our new blockbuster statin* [cholesterol-lowering drug] *should be called? The 5 best brand-names will win an Apple iShuffle* (valued, when I looked at a catalogue, at around $300). Checking the Medicines Australia code of practice I was interested to read section 3.7 which deals with prizes permitted in competitions. The money value is a matter of individual discretion, but "prizes which might be useful in the practice of medicine but are not specific to medicine or pharmacy must not be offered."

At one of the pharmacies where I once worked, the Arrow rep was a young friendly father of two who remembered all our names and always brought cakes. I enjoyed his visits and used to enquire after his children. He left the company before I began my research for this essay, so I wrote a polite email to the PR officer of Arrow, asking for an interview and setting out some of my questions.

Perhaps I shouldn't have been surprised, yet I was (based, naively, on my easy relationship with the former rep) when I received a return phone call from another staffer (not the PR man) who spoke to me in a manner that bordered on hostile. He caught me on my mobile while I was driving and I asked a minute's grace while I pulled off the road. Being away from my desk without pen or paper, I attempted to set up an interview at another time, flagging that my line of enquiry would be patents and cross-licencing. His phone manner, which had been glacial at the start, shifted into another register. I've heard that tone before. It's an unmistakeable human noise with overtones of the warning growl peculiar to canines. Rejoining the traffic, I made up my mind not to pursue the interview. The non-verbal content of his message had come through loud and clear.

It is the sound, I suspect, of drug company staffers rehearsing their back-off manoeuvres in preparation for filmmaker Michael Moore's investigation into the US pharmaceutical industry. Reporting in early 2005 on the forthcoming project, the *Sydney Morning Herald* printed this comment from a senior director in a US drug company lobby group: "We have an image problem not only with Michael Moore but with the general public. We're put in the same category as the tobacco industry, even though we save lives."

Our own code of practice in Australia denies drug companies the right to advertise their prescription-only products on television. Specifically: "Promotion of prescription-only products to the general public is prohibited by law." For this prohibition we must feel ourselves blessed.

The FDA gave approval for Direct to Customer or DTC advertising in 1997 and American television programming is now punctuated with frequent commercials for drugs whose names we only know here through doctor–patient contact. DTC advertising is expensive: Glaxo reportedly paid $91 million for Paxil [Aropax] TV ads in 2001, more than Nike spent on its top-of-the-range shoes.

I asked my friends on Long Island NY to report back to me on the frequency and kinds of ads they saw on evening broadcasts. They listed products for erectile dysfunction, arthritis, herpes, depression, birth control, allergy, nail fungus, asthma, advertised over two nights. "All these ads feature average and/or attractive people who are having a much better lifestyle because of their meds. Towards the end of the ad there is a rapidly spoken disclaimer about possible side effects." I'm reminded of Elizabeth Wurtzel's cry from the heart that serious conditions were being trivialised by media playfulness during the peak madness period of the people's love affair with Prozac (for example, *Rolling Stone* calling Prozac "the hot yuppie upper"): "a state of mind once considered tragic has become completely commonplace, even worthy of comedy." Perhaps this is what happens when we strip away the mystery, when in the rush to know everything, to conquer every barrier to human inquiry, we convert complex concepts into pixels and serious illness into a joke.

Because of the way it underlined the impact of DTC advertising, I was drawn to a "song" (really a rant set to music) played on the radio one day. Intrigued, I asked around: did anybody know the piece I was referring to, where the singer expresses his frustration at modern America, taking a swipe at obesity, homelessness, self-esteem, terrorist masterminds and drugs? "It's Lazyboy," I was told. The song is called "Underwear Goes inside the Pants". I found the lyrics on the internet. Here is the second verse:

> You know we have more prescription drugs now.
> Every commercial that comes on TV is a prescription drug ad.

I can't watch TV for four minutes without thinking I have five
    serious diseases.
Like: "Do you ever wake up tired in the morning?"
Oh my god, I have this, write this down. Whatever it is, I have it.
Half the time I don't even know what the commercial is:
People running in fields or flying kites or swimming in the ocean.
I'm like: that is the greatest disease ever. How do you get that?
That disease that comes with a hot chick and a puppy.

The burden of treating depression is carried by general practitioners, who if they are over forty years old have had to learn about SSRIs on the job. "It's a tough role," Dr T., a psychiatrist, told me. "GPs are the gateway through which troubled people have to pass if they want medical help." Dr T. spoke to me from a call centre where she answers telephone enquiries from GPs about psychiatric issues. She has a private practice and is also an attending specialist at a hospital. "People who can't deal with their lives, or solve their problems, become anxious and depressed and end up in the doctor's office. As I said, it's a tough role."

In my own small survey of general practice I visited six GPs and spoke to two more by telephone. I recorded the stories of eight good people doing the hard work of primary care.

All but the most recently qualified doctor had experienced a revolution in their understanding of the term "depression" since their "psych rotation" term as an intern. All had seen the extreme end of the depressive spectrum – the hospitalised, suicidal, sometimes catatonic patients – and all agreed that this type of patient rarely presented to a general practice doctor. Those who trained in the '70s and '80s emerged from their education with ideas about depression which they now believed were redundant and counterproductive. One male doctor, Dr M., had started out with the notion that depression was a kind of moral weakness that could be overcome with an improved attitude and meaningful work.

Dr M.'s early understanding of depression was shaped in part by the moral values (including reward through suffering) of the generation preceding his. His own generation, the baby boomers, kept this flame alive to a certain extent as they aged, engaging in a search for meaning in life by following the narrative of their own unfolding days, going back to look at bends in the road to wonder if they might have done things better, or been wiser in their choices, and ultimately feeling unsettled in the new, rapidly changing world of the twenty-first century. Initially, the baby boomers were the group most outraged by the Prozac revolution, and the most vocal in condemning prescription drugs that promised an easy detour around the rites of passage they had been forced to stumble through.

Dr M. no longer thinks that depression is a moral weakness. He is confident that depression is an organic disease and he has successfully treated hundreds of patients with SSRIs. He feels he has a firm grip on what depression looks and sounds like, and the way to turn it around by the "drugs first, talk later" approach. His approach, he assures me, is not mechanistic, just practical. Dr M. uses SSRIs initially, "then when they can listen" he introduces adjunct therapies. He gives long consultations and employs "fake it until you make it" tactics, telling his patients to "behave as though you have energy". He is scrupulous in following up.

Dr G. characterised the shift in his understanding of depression differently. In his early years he imagined depression as an entity with uniform traits and a textbook treatment. Twenty-five years into general practice he is infinitely more attuned to the complexities and idiosyncrasies of the beast. Now practising in a geographical area with a higher than normal suicide rate he has undertaken extra training to help him detect the at-risk patient. To this end he is mindful of seizing the moment. He starts his patients on drugs "to restore the chemical imbalance" and makes safety contracts, giving some patients his mobile number, making appointment dates two days ahead, constructing (sometimes from nothing) a "system of safety" to support them through a dark passage. Dr G.'s Eastern European background has imbued him with a respect for "hearing the story" and he maintains "a continuity of listening" while keeping a clinician's eye on the bodily expressions of deep unhappiness.

When I asked both doctors if they thought antidepressants were overprescribed, Dr M. dismissed the claim as an over-reaction. He hopes that the figure of a 58 per cent growth in antidepressant prescribing in the past four years will continue to climb as people become more confident in bringing their symptoms to a doctor. Dr G. put his answer in the context of the limits on a general practice visit. He has read the evolutionary psychology theorists and has been following the public debate about the over-use of drugs, but in the end he is faced with a patient in the chair and a finite consultation time. He will do whatever it takes to get his patient well.

There was such a shared-world, pro-drug view within my small sample that coming upon Dr H. required an adjustment in my approach. Dr H. runs a holistic practice and does not prescribe antidepressants. He has never seen any convincing proof that "depression is caused by a deficiency of SSRIs." His clientele is radically different from the norm. "Like seeks like," he says, so the people who come to him are not looking for a quick fix, nor is he offering one. His take on the depression phenomenon is based on adrenal exhaustion and his regime involves dialogue, vitamins, detoxification, rehydration and nutrient supplements. Far from taking a position in the debate, he rejects its very existence. New drugs don't interest him, he hasn't seen a drug rep since medical school, and drug company pervasiveness happens, as far as he is concerned, in another world.

Dr E. left her comfortable Sydney suburban practice eighteen months ago to work in the Northern Territory at an Aboriginal women's health clinic. In the familiar setting of her old general practice ("mostly women, mostly smears and tears") she had prescribed antidepressants with confidence. She became as adept as most of her colleagues in negotiating the emotional hurdles with a judicious combination of talk, support and pharmacotherapy. "In the dominant white culture there is an expectation that says: 'I deserve to be happy.'" This grid, however, would not fit over her new medical life where obviously troubled indigenous women do not present "sobbing about feeling unhappy", and where the women do not have a vocabulary of well-practised "white" depression-speak. Dr E. sees numbers of women with significant reactive depressions associated with poverty, violence, powerlessness, substance abuse, sexually transmitted diseases and infertility.

"I accept all the studies on serotonin and noradrenaline and dopamine. They do affect mood, I've seen the results in my [Sydney] practice. But does it empower someone who lives out here to take an SSRI? No, it doesn't. When the baseline they're coming from is poverty and despair, when their bleakness is a reaction to bereavement from stolen generation stuff or kids hanging themselves in gaol or the high mortality rate from common diseases – addressing the social problems is where we have to start, not jiggling around a few chemicals in their brains. One of my patients has a lot of mental-health issues that would be treated aggressively by pharmacotherapy in Sydney, but up here she's working with traditional healers. Someone has stolen her spirit. That's the diagnosis. I don't feel in a position to argue. What am I going to do? Give her Zoloft and tell her to try some retail therapy?"

All general practitioners in my group estimated that up to 30 per cent of their clients were being treated for depression. All dismissed the notion that they were influenced by drug company representatives. Dr A. stated that she had a good rapport with her Pfizer rep and she often used the hand-outs which helped her patients towards an understanding of their (depressive) symptoms, but that all decisions were based on what was best for the individual patient. All doctors believed that patients on SSRIs needed to push through the start-up effects.

Dr S., the youngest in the sample, worked as a scientist for two years before taking up medical studies and is particularly critical of the data presented by drug reps. Uncritical acceptance of this data permeates the real world in which most practitioners move. There is no time to read the fine print, and even if there was, it is generally accepted that drug companies load the dice in favour of their product. They compare new drugs to placebos rather than existing drugs in the same group. They don't publish unfavourable results. They don't test for long enough, or on people who represent the real end-users of the product. Dr S. scrutinises wash-out times, and test parameters, and this helps her decide if the newest SSRI is as good as is claimed, but it has not turned her away from prescribing antidepressants. She sees about three patients a day who come in with mild depression, and a large number of young mothers with post-natal depression. "There is a community expectation of a quick fix and we have to deal with that. Patients don't want the hard slog [of psychotherapy], they want a prescription for, I guess you could say, happiness. I can't guarantee that. I'm a go low, go slow girl and I'm not in a hurry to write a script, but I will and I do."

When the prescriptions fail, or the case has complications, patients are referred on to psychiatrists like Dr T., who sees "lots of twenty to fifty-year-old women". At this level, her job is to assess the patient again from scratch, confirm the diagnosis, identify any barriers to getting well, and look for co-existing medical conditions that might be clouding the waters.

Occasionally she has to tell one of her patients that she isn't depressed at all. "They're mortified. Their expectations have been set up by having an appointment made with a specialist and they come in expecting a label to be put on their condition." I wondered what drove people to want a label. "Often, they're reluctant to accept that the difficulties lie with themselves, with the way they manage (or don't manage). Life isn't working for them so they want someone in authority to say it's not working because they're sick. Struggling people want that to be the answer."

During this period of rapid social change, the patient has begun to exert a small but telling influence in the consultation room. Knowledge of drugs and the basics of diagnosis via the internet have created a new breed of medical auto-didact. The layman has become articulate in the vocabulary and nuances of the depression culture.

There was a time when even the educated patient deferred to the doctor's authority: you took in your symptoms and waited for a pronouncement. Now, anyone with a computer and a bit of curiosity can locate papers on what's hot in neuropsychiatry and women's issues. I have a friend who has been struggling with menopause. She recently went to see her GP and said, with the authority of a keen reader, "I think we've moved beyond the realm of oestrogen deficiency, I think we're talking serotonin now." Thirty minutes later she left with a prescription for Lexapro, a new SSRI.

Not since the first English translations of Freud's work has the lay public become so fluent in depression-speak. The vocabulary of depressive behaviour and thinking rolls off our tongues as if each of us studied the disease at medical school. It has crept up on us, but if we pay attention we will hear and read and even utter from our own mouths the telling borrowed phrases.

Citizens who use Google to find out more about their prescribed SSRIs quickly meet serotonin on their computer screens – there were 1,920,000 links the last time I looked.

Serotonin, once unheard of outside inner sanctums of learning, hopped over the ivy-covered wall in the mid-1980s and has been wandering abroad ever since. I have been at backyard BBQs where this runaway word has partied in unusual places. Having one's serotonin level adjusted fits so many social metaphors: adjusting the mix in a carburettor, for instance – too rich and you flood the motor; too thin and you stall. Or, as an interviewee told me, too little and you are "good for nothing but playing Nirvana on repeat in a darkened bedroom".

Within a few years we had the language we'd apparently been hunting for: the way to say "I feel down" without sounding like an ageing hippy. This vocabulary, no longer the privilege of the psychiatrically trained, empowered us in dubious ways: we could now sentence ourselves without benefit of a medical judge; we began to speak of our genetic predispositions, black thoughts, flat affect, sense of alienation, suicidal ideation, obsessive-compulsive tendencies, even "touches of Asperger's", and the ubiquitous ADD and ADHD — all lifted out of their contexts and mixed into a lolly bag of useful jargon.

The professionals at the coalface (most often the prescribing doctor and the dispensing pharmacist) cannot afford to fall behind the new wised-up patient who has googled her symptoms and possible cures, and feels comfortable challenging the divide between "lay" knowledge and professional knowledge. Older doctors, a recent Harvard study tells us, are not always keeping up with the quick-march of technology and drug therapies. They're accused of being out of touch, and of being "more adept at humanistic rather than technical" approaches to disease.

What if all of us, in small ways, are contributing to the depression industry through the simple means of appropriating its language? Blame the cinema or television if you like. Or the internet.

We must at least question the potential damage we may do by shaping our doctors' visits. Just as a parent thinks she is in control of a helpless infant, it soon becomes apparent that though helpless, the child is forming the adult, eliciting responses to serve its own needs. And so it is with us, if we go in saying, as my friend did: "I have a serotonin problem." How do you know that you do? Where did your information come from? Your friend who feels better on Efexor? The internet? A TV documentary? Oprah? Browsing through the *DSM-IV*? Are we outsmarting ourselves and our own true needs?

Much of the debate about how to treat depression circles around the supposed impasse between talking therapies and drug therapies: the Freudian way versus the primacy of the brain chemicals. We as consumers have followed these two lines of thought informally through the medium of television and films (principally American), and along the way our patterns of usage have been changed and enlarged, often by humour.

Woody Allen taught us how to negotiate and enunciate our neuroses. In the film *Annie Hall*, Alvy Singer (played by Allen) is a fifteen-year veteran of psychoanalysis. "I'm giving it one more year," he says, "and then I'm going to Lourdes."

Nightly, Australian viewers tune into American sitcoms where dysfunctional family and social dynamics are dealt with in a sea of clever words and one-liners. Repeated exposure is, I believe, making a difference to the way we externalise (by way of speech and mannerisms) concerns that were once locked away from public view. We may learn, for instance, how to verbalise our social obsessions from such comedies. In *Seinfeld*, the humour, which stems from perceived dangers (embarrassment, rejection) in trivial situations (being sneered at by salesmen, the perils of bringing a gift to a dinner party) operates within the psychology of shame, a rich area of study for psychiatrists and shame-sensitive lay people who see the *Seinfeld* cast (and therefore themselves) exposed to the very forms of public torment they dread. Authors John D. Ratey and Catherine Johnson describe *Seinfeld* as "virtually a textbook of mild obsessive-compulsive disorder". None of the depicted social catastrophes results in profound levels of loss or rejection, as they do for instance in the higher-order phobias; rather the mild OCD sufferer becomes a "social scanner", constantly on the alert for the *faux pas*.

> *Kramer*: Ah, what kind of a man are you? The guy is unconscious in
>   a coma and you don't have the guts to kiss his girlfriend?
> *Jerry*: I didn't know what the coma etiquette was.

Unconsciously we learn from such exchanges. Mild OCD is on the rise in Australia and social phobia is an approved condition for SSRI prescribing. Even if the connection is a slender one, there are issues worth pondering as we ask ourselves how we come to know what we know, and consider the possible repercussions of playfully labelling ourselves and our friends with psychological tags.

Angie, twenty-two, had been self-harming (with a razor blade) since she was fourteen. In her first serious relationship she lived with a partner who was on Aropax "and open about it". It was Angie's first experience of someone being medicated. She saw the side effects (often resulting from inconsistent compliance – missing doses then doubling up), and the terrible withdrawal effects her partner endured after stopping, cold turkey.

When Angie was twenty and at university (and out of the relationship), she became moody and despairing – "I wasn't truly suicidal, I'm a bit snobby about that, not having made my mark on the world yet" – and began self-harming again. Two weeks before an important event she saw a bulk-billing doctor close to campus (she chose a bulk-biller because she could "get in and out quickly") and said: "Just dose me up." The doctor gave her a free sample of Zoloft, explained the start-up effects, "said all the right things," and had her make a follow-up appointment. At home she went onto the internet: "I wanted to understand what I was putting into my body." She found "a whole bunch of rubbish, drug company-sponsored ads, and some mildly useful medical information". At the second appointment she committed to taking Zoloft for a year, but after two months she had a recurrence of the old anxieties, a dispiriting lack of concentration ("I was so vague") and a return of the desire to self-harm. Her doctor advised her to "push through", stop drinking and smoking dope, get more sleep, "or she would put me on Aropax". Having been through the Aropax experience with her former partner (perceived by both of them as a negative one), she took stock. "Then I got a good job, a really good job where people looked up to me and that was the impetus. I still get down, I still *feel* it but I can't *show* it. And no more carving marks on my arms, people notice that sort of thing."

Angie also uses recreational drugs like ecstasy "as a treat, about once a month". And speed sometimes when she wants a buzz. "How", I asked, "does she reconcile her ambivalence about Zoloft with the risk of party drugs that could come from anywhere or contain anything?" (This, I realise, is my own baby-boomer incredulity speaking.)

"When I was at high school we used to buy Ritalin off kids with ADD. But it's such a clean medicated *exact* dose. I mean what were we doing? I don't really care about bad outcomes in a social setting now with E and speed, it's something I know how to deal with, but getting into this *Valley of the Dolls* thing, popping pills every day to balance out my brain chemistry, it seems so institutionalised. It's the cheque-book analogy thing. Have I spent it all? Should I top up?"

Had she tried any of the accepted non-drug approaches, analysis or cognitive behaviour therapy or counselling?

"Therapy is for self-obsessed freaks," she said. "If I hear about another life spiral or dream plan I'll throttle someone."

Angie had read *Prozac Nation*, the iconic first-person account of Elizabeth Wurtzel's battle with depression and her experience of Prozac when that drug was new and quite unknown. In the epilogue to the book, Wurtzel wrestles with the SSRI phenomenon:

> I have no way to be certain of this, but my guess is that most people on Prozac haven't taken the circuitous path to the drug that I did … By the time I was put on Prozac they'd tried everything else possible, I'd had my brain fried and blunted with so many other drugs, I'd spent over a decade in a prolonged state of clinical despair. Nowadays, Prozac seems to be a panacea available for the asking.

Wurtzel and Angie, born ten years apart in a generation that is resigned to upheaval – is, in fact, comfortable in upheaval – insist on constructing a mental illness narrative that is uniquely their own, one that accepts the role of serotonin-boosting antidepressant drugs while rejecting any victim labels or angst about the big bad changing world. Wurtzel circles in on her theme when she tries to think of alternatives:

The trouble is that when we get around to solutions, it always seems to come down to Prozac. Or Zoloft or Paxil. Deep clinical depression is a disease, one that not only can, but probably should, be treated with drugs. But a low-grade terminal anomie, a sense of alienation or disgust or detachment, the collective horror at a world that seems to have gone so very wrong, is not a job for anti-depressants.

Another interviewee, Susan, thirty-five, rejected the drug route even though it was offered:

> I have been quite depressed in the past, but I managed to stumble through without [antidepressant drugs]. I luckily found a wonder-ful holistic GP and counsellor who helped me through it and I think, for me, it was strengthening to discover my own resources (somehow for me I felt taking medication would confirm my "madness"). I soon discovered, with her help, that what I assumed was a permanent state of being for me, was something grounded in real events that I could eventually come to terms with. Since then I've never been depressed like that again (and I was sure it would recur all my life).

In follow-up correspondence, Susan reflected on her decision:

> I had to absolutely trust my GP and it was hard (one member of my family was particularly pushy about my need for antidepressants) but it was worth persisting with taking a different approach. I often wonder if I had taken the drugs if I would feel a desperate need to go back on them anytime I felt myself feeling low; instead now I sit with it [her depression] for a bit and I can usually find a reason for feeling that way and deal with it before it gets out of hand. I think this approach works for reactive depression but perhaps is less effective for the really entrenched forms of depression.

The contrast between younger people with mild to moderate depression and their grandparents who suffer varying forms of geriatric depression lights up in exchanges that take place across the counters of pharmacies, where both groups sign for their drugs. From my vantage point I see a kind of unquestioning acceptance of drug therapies among the younger group, and, at times, a deeply troubled response from the older group, who struggle with a heritage of meeting challenges with courage and accepting unhappiness as part of the mix.

It is wounding for older citizens to face the prospect that no one needs them anymore. It is sad and (yes) depressing, but, they ask, is a drug the answer?

In 1956, Linus Pauling and others predicted that it would only be a matter of time before mental disorders would be found to have their causes in biochemical and genetic bases. This is a scientific attitude that rests on the assumption that human behaviour may be adequately explained by organic theories, and it is the launching pad for most of the medical breakthroughs in modern times.

The incorporation of dominantly scientific goals into medical pioneering has been both a blessing and a vexation. The blessings are obvious: we know more facts. But what is vexing is the advancement of knowledge at the sacrifice of medicine's true north pole, health.

Illness, in another time, was understood in terms of man's connection to his external world and all its infringing forces; the stars, the planets, the sun, the moon, the seasons, the tides, even the hut in which he shared food with his family. One of the nuisances of the scientific revolution has been an alteration to this wider cosmic perspective. The world, instead of being out there, has been subsumed inside the human vehicle. We have become our own worlds. Medical explorers delve into the human body's flesh and blood and grey matter sure that all the answers lie hidden in the cellular cities and suburbs. This continual narrowing of the gaze, long acknowledged to be dehumanising, has emphasised the micro at the expense of the macro. It partly explains our delight with the word "selective" in the context of a brain-altering drug. But put the word "selective" in front of the word "school" and you get a sense of elitism. In a medical context, selectivity leads us on like a beckoning hand. The answer to depression is here, the sign says, in the synaptic cleft.

Lived experience, a life story moving through a landscape peopled with family and friends and colleagues, and framed by hierarchies often beyond our control, has little place in the clinical trials upon which decisions to license a drug are made. Rigorous evidence-based outcome studies are not set up for nuance.

William Blake called this continual peering down a microscope looking for answers "single vision". Similarly in the forward striving movement of allopathic, or drug-based, medicine, the perspective seems to have narrowed to one sharp point: to refine, to particularise, to achieve the holy grail of scientific endeavour − smart-bomb accuracy.

Dr Candace B. Pert, co-discoverer of serotonin binding receptors, wrote a letter to the editor of *Time* magazine in October 1997:

> I am alarmed at the monster that John Hopkins neuroscientist Solomon Snyder and I created when we discovered the simple binding assay for drug receptors 25 years ago … The public is being misinformed about the precision of these selective serotonin uptake inhibitors when the medical profession oversimplifies their action in the brain and ignores the body as if it merely exists to carry the head around!

At a recent convention of psychiatrists who gathered to consider alternative approaches to treating mental illness, there was a rebel cry from inside the ranks:

> Mainstream psychiatry is now limited to a radical materialist ideology whereby the human subject is seen as a bag of chemicals that we can do clever titrations with; we should be less subservient to drug companies' vested interests, and esteem moment to moment felt experience.

After a relapse into depression and an attempted suicide after several months on Prozac, the wonder cure, Elizabeth Wurtzel noted that:

> Mental health is so much more complicated than any pill that any mortal can invent … Just as many germs have outsmarted antibiotics … so depression manages to reconfigure itself so that it is more than just a matter of too little serotonin … I believe, perhaps superstitiously … that brain cells will always outsmart medical

molecules. If you are chronically down, it is a lifelong fight to keep from sinking.

William Styron booked himself into a hospital just in time. Others sink. About 15 per cent of major depressions proceed to suicide. Some end their lives on the end of a noose in a park at night. Or in a gas oven with babies upstairs asleep.

No illness state has one form of treatment that is applicable and accurate for all. Alcohol and illegal drugs have been the traditional self-administered antidote to unhappiness since antiquity. In *The Anatomy of Melancholy*, Maginus recommends getting drunk "once a month at least … because it scours the body by vomit, urine, sweat, of all manner of super-fluities, and keeps it clean". Other authorities speak of the benefits of opium, datura, and "a posset of hemp seed", all still popular, all proven evasive tactics for numbing and anaesthetising psychic pain.

The rise of psychology and its uptake into wider society since the 1950s has fashioned the way we understand our lives and identity. We evaluate our progress using psychology's language and measure our success against its norms.

If we don't measure up on, say, an attitude or mood scale, we may be offered the option of correcting our deviation through analysis (the long way) or a mood-altering drug (the shorter way) or both. We have choices. We may choose a posset of hemp seed and simply opt out of the medical model. We may enter psychoanalysis and begin a long dialogue with our behaviours. But if we choose SSRIs, we are demonstrating our preparedness to seek out drugs to shape our identities; we are complicit in acknowledging our bodies as faulty machines that can be fixed bio-chemically.

We need help, of course, to arrive at this point. First we have to enter the consulting room and participate in a clinical discourse. Two person-alities, the doctor and the patient, have to talk to each other. If a disorder is diagnosed, the nature of clinical discourse is such that it becomes almost impossible for either the physician or the patient to consider or even imagine an "elsewhere" beyond the zone in which disorders attract cures.

It has been argued that a prescription for a mood-altering drug reduces the necessity for the patient to come to terms with past behaviour. What happened in the time leading up to taking a seat in the doctor's office becomes redundant. The future becomes the target. The time starts from now, when the first tablet is swallowed. By choosing to claim a depressive identity, we turn away from the past and – in our own meek way – contribute to the new collective avoidance of taking responsibility for our own lives.

This is another way of saying that the Prozac-style drugs swept aside the older, "modernist" view that depression was a pathway to identity.

Let us retreat a few steps here, to what is claimed for SSRIs. Given that we prescribe these drugs for high-school students, it might benefit us to go back into the high-school science classroom and reacquaint ourselves with the basics of this complex system called neurotransmission.

The depressed brain looks like any other brain, "as big as a coconut, the colour of uncooked liver, the consistency of chilled butter". But at a cellular level, specifically the 10 per cent of brain cells that are adapted to carry electrical signals (the neurons), there is a glitch. At each connection point, in the tiny gap called the synapse across which electrical signals move, it is postulated that some of the fifty different neurotransmitters which facilitate the passage of signals from one neuron to another are not there in sufficient quantity, or are being mopped up or deactivated by enzymes. The most studied, and so far considered to be most important, of these chemical messengers are dopamine, serotonin and noradrenaline.

At a macro level, brain imaging purports to show the consequences of not having enough serotonin for prolonged periods: parts of the frontal lobes become drastically underactive. There is only a dim glow from the areas that make us want to get up and get going, or pay attention to the outside world, or make plans for the future (our self-willed actions). In contrast to this low voltage output, there are areas of overactivity: the parts that hold onto long-term memories and negative feelings. Joining these are relay stations and neural pathways so that when something fires up the circuit, the loop activates and the depressive cycle begins.

Serotonin and dopamine are part of a complex circuit that helps to shape human behaviour, and the message is that increased serotonin is good for the brain's chemical balance. To achieve this increase we can interfere with the natural metabolism of serotonin by blocking the enzyme which zaps it, or take over-the-counter supplements: "natural" serotonins from plants, or chemical precursors in the serotonin pathway.

This model is common to many deficiency syndromes, decreased bone density in osteoporosis, for instance, which is treated by taking in added calcium through the diet or in tablet form, or by interfering with the removal of old bone with drugs like Fosamax.

The strongest opponents of SSRIs have attempted to make a case for widespread societal changes following two generations of Prozac use. The US International Coalition for Drug Awareness, for instance, links the increase in anti-social behaviours (impulsivity, hostility, addiction) to the high uptake by millions of American citizens of drugs that convert serotonin levels when there is some doubt that an adjustment is required or appropriate (e.g. in cases of mild to moderate depression). Given that altered serotonin levels are also found in psychotic and schizophrenic states they argue that we (society) should question the medical system which allows so many people access to serotonin-boosting drugs.

A lot of ratbag ideas about serotonin and neurotransmitters circulate on the internet. Hedweb.com is worth a visit to read its abstract on the Hedonistic Imperative, a manifesto for eradicating suffering in all sentient life. Whereas the Coalition fears mass antisocial behaviour by humans doped up on Zoloft, this site encourages all people to go into "dopamine-overdrive" in order to enhance "exploratory and goal-directed activity".

I point out these extremes for obvious reasons. When science itself in all its sophistication and striving for excellence can't be absolutely sure about the correctness of its hypothesis on the actions of mood-altering drugs, we as consumers are unlikely to stumble across the answers by surfing the net.

The result of reading from good and bad sources can, however, be detected in the high rate of placebo responses to SSRIs in developed countries today.

In a 2002 study of the six most widely prescribed antidepressants, based on forty-two drug company-audited clinical trials, placebos were found to be 80 per cent as effective as SSRIs and their variants. Within the trials there were individual variations (high response to nil response), but the averaged figures suggest a poor showing from the much-hyped mood stabilisers, and also highlight the amount of drug company spin that has to be applied to sex up the results.

Individual practitioners have also been publishing studies that cast doubt on the effectiveness of SSRIs (for example a paper from Massachusetts General Hospital concluding that only 30 to 40 per cent of people taking SSRIs get a high-quality response, while others get a partial or incomplete response, or no response at all), but their voices, it seems, have been lost in the popular clamour.

Seen in this light, the new generation of antidepressants no longer appear to be the miracle drugs we were led to believe. And yet, doctors and patients all around the country continue to praise them to the skies. "I wouldn't go as far as saying put SSRIs in the drinking water," said one GP, "but I'm tempted."

"I can still remember reading about the workings of neurotransmitters in the library – it was their almost mechanical working that was fascinating then. The day I got my prescription for Cipramil I felt this frisson of joy, and I hadn't even started taking the pills. I knew about the placebo effect with SSRIs and I was hoping if the drug didn't take the placebo effect would, a sort of placebo's placebo." I received these words in an email from a friend now living in Uganda. "The changes wrought, though, were not only beyond my expectations, they were beyond what I imagined could be wrought."

Simply by weighing up the pros and cons of medicating depression, overhearing conversations about successes and failures, and becoming familiar with the names of pharmaceuticals, we enter a state of mental preparedness for the arrival of an antidepressant into our own lives.

This expectation factor poses an interesting question about the effectiveness of SSRIs. Do they work because of a pre-existing mind-set for success in the consumer; do they work *regardless* of the mind-set and experience of the consumer; do they work full-stop?

It seems, from recent studies, that if the patient has some knowledge about the intended outcome of therapy before they begin (as was the case with my correspondent) a part of their brain unrelated to the drug target-site lights up. Activity can be detected with brain scanning within a week of the good news. The area that lights up is the *expectation area*, a site linked to rewards and formerly thought to be only associated with addiction.

The shaping idea that you have a chemical imbalance that can be fixed by taking a drug acts like a pro-drug itself, a softener that sets up a smoother process towards getting better.

Cognitive behaviour therapy (CBT) also targets a pathway to recovery in the brain, but along a completely different route. The target is in the cortex, the thinking part of the brain which can reconfigure problem-solving and the way we react to stress. The current consensus is that a combination of drug and CBT produces better results than drug alone, with help coming from two unrelated but compatible sources.

The placebo rate in the developed world has increased noticeably since the 1960s, a phenomenon that can be related directly to the psychologisation of our language and the ease with which we now speak openly about our anxieties and depressions. Where sufferers were once isolates, communicating their anguish to a spouse or doctor with little or no expectation of relief in the future, the taboo subject of depression and all its euphemisms has gone public.

Science has put a lot of energy into elucidating depression's intricacies, right down to the level of chemicals in small gaps in our brain. Psychiatry has addressed the destructive patterns of negative thinking. Therapists have devised step-wise plans for breaking cycles of wrong thinking. And the internet-connected, newspaper-reading, documentary-watching public engages continuously with the flow of information. When science gets it wrong and self-corrects, we hear about it, and accept (even admire) examples of apparent fortitude in the face of tricky obstacles. Around this public spectacle, staged like a battle (we are *fighting* depression), is a smog of dashed hopes and flashing particles of insight from which the lay person divines an expectation that help is on the way. This is the placebo effect.

The patients who don't tune in to these battle cries have low placebo rates. Indigenous Australians in outback communities, for instance. Urban patients whose depression has not yielded to drug therapy, or has yielded then crashed, and left them on a treadmill of electro-convulsive therapy, hospitalisation, even surgery. As one professor of psychiatry put it: "These people have no expectation, in fact their placebo response is driving in the opposite direction, so you're fighting depression on two fronts, at least."

In developing countries the only SSRIs are found in the travelling bags of Western visitors or in private pharmacies for patients rich enough to pay. The World Health Organization has a list of 316 essential medicines approved for public expenditure, and in the category of "Medicines used for Mood Disorder" there is exactly one entry, amitriptyline tablet 25mg.

An argument for fewer drugs, not more, was put forward by Dr Robert Moulds, Professor of Medicine at the Fiji School of Medicine, Suva, in an editorial in *Australian Prescriber* entitled "Expensive new drugs – do we really need them?" He attacks the "article of faith" that in modern medicine we need new drugs because old drugs are "old", less efficient, less specific. On this logic, developing countries are handicapped by a lack of access to the latest and greatest. Not so, writes Dr Moulds. "We can treat most conditions perfectly adequately with the older drugs available on the essential drugs list." Of course there are exceptions. There is no "statin" for patients with cardiovascular disease, and there are no anti-retroviral drugs for AIDS patients. Diabetic clients don't have the new oral hypoglycaemics, but, writes Dr Moulds, "our woefully poor control of diabetes is mainly caused by socio-economic factors rather than lack of access to newer drugs."

Dr Moulds is really arguing with the PBS system in Australia, which rewards pharmaceutical companies with patent protection (that is, protection against competition) for new drugs that are neither truly innovative nor essential to health. Patent protection also applies to drugs which

Dr Moulds believes represent "trivial developments". He reminds us that the PBS came into being "when most new drugs, such as penicillin, were truly life-saving, but unaffordable to most people."

"Depression" in my father's time meant saving string and turning off electric lights. Modern medicine pretends that depression is a disease of the late twentieth century, responsive only to the newest miracles of neuroscience. I want to suggest that this new thing "depression" is not new at all. Depression is what depression has always been, not a recently identified opportunistic virus like AIDS but a cluster of symptoms that signal a deeper, more complex malaise. Nor is it homogeneous in its appearance or expression, or unanimously responsive to drug therapies. Some depressions are deadly. Severely depressed people need all the help they can get; they need drugs and psychotherapies and hospitals and expert nurturing.

Other forms are mild and self-limiting. A holiday or a receptive friend may be all that is required to nurse a sad person through a bad patch.

For the in-between group, the answers are less clear-cut. Mild to moderately depressed people need something more sustaining than a week on a tropical beach or extended coffee mornings. But what are we, realistically, to do for this large amorphous group? The medical response has been to give them drugs and counselling, with the accent on drugs. Only 15 per cent of mild to moderately depressed people go to someone other than a doctor for help; the majority seek their answers from medicine via science.

Depression is still a mystery to science, even now. Medical treatment is predicated on the idea that we know and understand depression's causes. There may be cause to wonder if we are swallowing our Zoloft and Efexor to stave off psychic pain in a sort of parody of our string-saving forebears; doing something, however problematic, because it is more than doing nothing.

As depression edges forward as our number one health burden in the developed world, the quest for solutions exercises scientists in predictable ways: they are digging even deeper into the tissues and cells of human life, going where no one has been before, submerging past the limits of former deep exploration. They are shining their torches on our genes.

Genomics, the newest untapped oilfield, will yield up more drugs to mask unhappiness, and the news is already out. The World Health Organization estimates that there are currently 500 targets for drug therapy; a figure that could increase ten-fold as the territory of the human genome is explored and mapped. The guiding principle behind much of this work is the search for biochemical pathways that lead to a deficiency or over-supply of some chemical or enzyme. Once identified, the task is to interfere with a key component in the sequence of events, thereby correcting the irregularity. The correcting chemical is then refashioned into a tablet, trialled and if approved and PBS listed, will appear in a pharmacy near you in about ten years' time. We can almost certainly look forward to a finessing of the serotonin model of depression.

"Serotonin was kind of sexy for a while," Dr K., a psychiatrist in hospital practice told me. "Now we have neurotransmitters one or two levels up from that. The drugs are getting pretty sophisticated."

During a recent airing of the public-health issues around SSRI over-prescribing in the UK, reported by BBC News, the urgent need for more non-drug resources – which was taken as read by mental-health charities like Rethink and Sane, and welcomed by The Royal College of Physicians – was coolly received by drug companies. "New guidance clarifies the use of such drugs," a spokesman said, "but it has to be remembered that SSRIs have revolutionised the treatment of depression."

For people suffering chronic unresolved depression, attacking the technology that might one day deliver peace of mind seems mean-spirited and unhelpful. "Counselling and exercise are a lame panacea for a very real malady," a correspondent wrote in response to the BBC program. There are obviously things that are right and good about scientific research, and there is room in this discussion to admire and praise discoveries. Major depression, it can't be stated often enough, requires a major intervention. But if the quest is to be democratic we need to restore some of the complexity to our portrait of depression – we need to admit that there is more to mental health than neural goal-kicking.

The more difficult challenge asks us to address our confusion about what constitutes happiness.

Realistically, happiness-recovery can't be the mandate of general practitioners, the group of professionals who are at the frontline of patient access, says psychiatrist Dr K.: "GPs don't have 50 minutes to get at the fundamentals and help re-frame a world view."

In Australia, GPs can now refer a patient for up to six Medicare-funded sessions with a psychologist. But the system has its limits and frustrations. When the six visits are up, where does the patient turn? $175 for a one-hour session with a psychologist in private practice is too much to pay for most wage earners, but what about $35 for a book? Is this the way forward?

A quick tour of bookstores and bestseller lists shows a flourishing self-help trade. When a particular book hits the mark with a reader, there can be a sense that the words are personalised and affirming. Bibliotherapy has become a kind of lay religion for some, with the appeal of a one-on-one accord that bypasses a mediating vicar or health professional.

In the UK, the National Health Service (NHS) is providing "Books on Prescription" in two pilot schemes in Cardiff and Devon. The trial is in its early days and will be watched with both friendly interest and scepticism.

It came about as a response to new NHS guidelines which encourage psychological treatments over drug treatments in the early stages of mild to moderate depression. GPs co-operating in the experiment have the option of referring a mildly depressed patient to a self-help clinic where the patient is given a reading list and presumably reports back to the mental-health officer as they progress through the texts. There is a retro-feel to this worthy project. I'm reminded of the days when a good bookstore employee knew his stock and his customers and could match you up with the exact book able to light up your day.

No such scheme is mooted for Australian patients. Psychologists remain unconvinced. Success depends too heavily on certain organising principles already fired up and operating in the depressed and seeking individual. The therapist's power to challenge wrong thinking is negated in the scenario of a patient working solo through a book. The advocates of drug therapies also doubt the value of "recipe books", especially when their patients have reduced powers of concentration and little recourse to self-willed gamesmanship.

At the top of many connoisseurs' reading lists on depression is William Styron's *Darkness Visible: A Memoir of Madness*. Right on the cusp of a major revolution in pharmacotherapy (one that would see Prozac appear on the cover of *Newsweek* and *New York* magazines and establish a publishing sub-category of books with Prozac in the title) Styron fell victim to two appalling life events: the onset of late-life major clinical depression, followed by and made worse by wrong-headed management by his physician.

As his nervous system spun out of control, he was put on Ativan, a tranquilliser from the benzodiazepine family. Given the staggeringly ill-considered medical advice that he could take Ativan "as casually as aspirin", Styron (who was exhausted by sleeplessness) gradually increased the dose to three times the recommended limit. His psychiatrist then started him on an outpatient course of maprotoline (Ludiomil), a new-generation tricyclic antidepressant which had disagreeable side effects, gave no relief and which Styron abandoned as his depression became markedly worse. (The psychiatrist apparently missed the author's suicidal thoughts or he would have bypassed the prescription and sent his patient straight to hospital.)

Desperate to escape into sleep (and, it soon became clear, its dark companion, death), Styron asked if there was anything better than Ativan to combat insomnia whereupon he was switched to the sweetly named Halcion which he also took at triple dose.

The crisis point was a self-recognition that he would suicide if he stayed at home and from the depths of anguish, he woke his wife. "I drew upon some last gleam of sanity to perceive the terrifying dimensions of the mortal predicament I had fallen into ... The next day I was admitted to hospital."

Halcion has been banned in some countries for its propensity to incite suicidal thinking in susceptible people. "One cringes", writes Styron, "when thinking about the damage such promiscuous prescribing of these potentially dangerous tranquillisers may be creating in patients everywhere." When he stopped taking Halcion, his suicidal thoughts "dwindled then disappeared".

In a strange way this indictment of one particular benzodiazepine (not, it should be noted, the tricyclic antidepressant, which had its own unwanted physical effects but did not incite a self-harming crisis) presages what would happen with the advent of Prozac. Many successful permanent exits from harrowing despair would accompany the introduction of SSRIs into depression therapy.

Styron credits his recovery (in part) to "sequestration" and "benign detention" in a hospital where "one's only duty is to get well."

Depression, however, is not always catastrophic. Sometimes it is gloomy without being impenetrably black, and sometimes it is quirky and involves phobias.

I am thinking of John Cheever's fine short story "The Angel on the Bridge" in which the narrator develops what seems to be a family tendency towards height phobias. At first exasperated by his mother who won't fly in aeroplanes and slightly disdainful of his older brother who is terrified in elevators, Cheever's storyteller suddenly succumbs to an irrational fear of driving over bridges. His symptoms, so familiar to phobics and trauma casualties, crackle on the page like errant lightning strikes, building ominously towards the big one, the one that will explode like a bomb and blow all to smithereens. The thing that saves him, the lightning rod that carries off all that damaging energy, is a chance meeting with a hitchhiker, a folk-singer carrying a harp (the angel of the title). Her ordinary kindness gets him over the bridge. Like the cognitively retrained brain, which has learnt to face fear with strategies, the folk-singer distracts the driver long enough for the car wheels to roll the distance to safe ground. This story might be a gift to put alongside a generic self-help book with a title like *Overcoming Depression*. Just a suggestion.

When William Styron writes, "For me the real healers were seclusion and time," I'm reminded of the work of Dorothy Rowe, who has written that depression is not an illness but a defence mechanism, a place to retreat to when things get too much.

A poet I correspond with sent me these lines of Rilke to think about ("something to ponder", she wrote) alongside the clinical trials and learned papers of depression theory.

> How we squander our hours of pain.
> How we gaze beyond them
> Into the bitter duration
> To see if they have an end
> Though they really are
> The seasons of us, our winter
>
> —Rainer Maria Rilke, "Tenth Duino Elegy"

My favourite guide-book through the terrain of mental suffering is *The Anatomy of Melancholy*. Never mind that it categorically avows that melancholy is caused by black bile, I don't care. The scientists will tug at depression's mysteries for years to come yet, and if they want to give primacy to a sexier neurotransmitter than serotonin and set off new gold rushes for the blocking enzyme, I will listen and marvel at their discoveries. Meanwhile, it is not wasted time to read old wisdom like this: "The manner of living is to more purpose than whatsoever can be drawn out of the most precious boxes of the apothecaries."

Here is melancholy's prescription, culled by Burton from the great writers of antiquity:

> Let the air be clear and moist most part: diet moistening, of good juice, easy of digestion, and not windy: drink clear [liquids], and well brewed, not too strong, nor too small. Exercise not too remiss, nor too violent. Sleep a little more than ordinary. Excrements daily to be voided by art or nature, avoid all passions and perturbations of the mind. Let him not be alone or idle but still accompanied with such friends and familiars he most affects, neatly dressed, washed, and combed, in clean sweet linen, spruce, handsome, decent, and good apparel.

The experts of the day were divided on the matter of blood-letting, but most practised it, though Burton himself "did hardly approve of this course".

What delights me is the recipe for sleep in the cure of melancholy:

> As waking, that hurts, by all means must be avoided, so sleep, which so much helps, by like ways must be procured, by nature or art, … and be protracted longer than ordinary … It moistens and fattens the body, concocts, and helps digestion, as we see in dormice, and those Alpine mice that sleep all winter, which Gesner speaks of, when they are found sleeping under the snow in the dead of winter, as fat as butter.

And on the value of friendship, quoting Seneca:

> It is the best thing in the world to get a trusty friend, to whom we may freely and sincerely pour out our secrets; nothing so delighteth and easeth the mind, as when we have a prepared bosom, to which our secrets may descend, of whose conscience we are assured as our own, whose speech may ease our succourless estate.

Even the more preposterous cures still have a certain kind of charm for a reader such as myself. I think of the egg, demonised by the cholesterol fascists in the '80s, having its moment of glory in the cure of melancholy. "After blood-letting we must proceed to other medicines; some of the chiefest I will rehearse. Rulandus' *absolute medicine* of 50 eggs, to be taken three in the morning."

CONTRAINDICATIONS

Figures seem to vary, but it is believed that one woman in fifteen and one man in thirty are affected by depression each year. Well over a million of our population are medicated daily for their affliction, be it mild or severe, and with each prescription there is an expectation (indeed a direction) that patients be warned of side effects. Not just at the start, but at a dosage change (up or down), and at the end, when tapering slowly is the only safe way to end a drug relationship.

Clearly not all the warning messages hit their targets, or make an impression lasting enough to keep our patients vigilant and alert. Or, as I hear over and over again, the message is never delivered in the first place.

There is a contentious issue at play in the matter of warnings. Ideally, it should be a three-part harmony. One voice each from the drug company (leaflet insert or box warning), the doctor (verbal plus hand-out) and the pharmacist (computer-printed leaflet and verbal, if desired by the patient).

As a pharmacist, I know that every drug has a warning list that would frighten any sane person into drug sobriety. This is why there are gradations in the level of information given. Judgments have to be made. From time to time it is necessary to venture into areas fraught with the dangers of too much information.

A lady I will call Fran brought me her son's prescription for Zoloft. A long-suffering mother aged sixty, Fran had been accompanying her son on the antidepressant merry-go-round while they waited for a psychiatric consultation (eight weeks and counting).

"Prozac", she told me, "did absolutely nothing. Efexor gave him humungous nightmares – he punched his bed so hard he bruised his knuckles. Avanza turned him into a zombie during the day and a raving loony at night." Efexor, the drug that seemed to work best in terms of relief from black moods and despair, also landed him with the most unmanageable side effects. "Humungous nightmares" can only be imagined.

"We got told nothing," she claims.

In the computer print-out I gave her, the common side effects of Zoloft are listed as: *nausea, nervousness, diarrhoea, constipation, headache, dry mouth, insomnia, restlessness, agitation, dizziness, sweating, drowsiness, fatigue, tremor, male sexual problems, and not wanting to eat.* Scanning the list, she said, unimpressed, "Oh, he's had all those, and more."

Under "Less Common Unwanted Effects", it read: *sensation of rapid heart beat, decrease or loss of touch or other senses, twitching, vomiting, fever, anxiety, yawning, female sexual problems, hot flushes, vision disturbance and seizures.*

Yet Zoloft, despite all its potential danger to mind and body, has been the most successful SSRI on the market for a decade because, according to the doctors who prescribe it and the majority of patients who take it, it has the best safety profile. "It works," said all of the doctors I interviewed (bar Dr H.). "I've watched it working for years, and I have confidence it will keep working."

For Fran's son, who must surely fall between stools in the SSRI game, I privately forecast more doom as I gave her the party line about her son pushing through the start-up side effects and calling his doctor if things got worse. I am not privy to the whole story. The pieces that concern drug side effects are the shards I am permitted to see. The whole broken pot is someone else's difficult mending task. As she signed for the Zoloft and left with only modest hopes that this was the miracle drug that would save her son, I hoped for swift progress in the queue towards the psychiatrist's couch, before something more terrible than drug side effects happened to him.

What about the children? In September 2004 the American FDA supported recommendations by the Psychopharmacologic Drugs and Pediatric Advisory Committee, and for the first time stated publicly that: "There is an increased risk of suicidality in pediatric patients, and the risk applies to all [antidepressant] drugs studied in the clinical trials." The committee recommended a black-box warning for use by children and teenagers, the provision of a patient information sheet to all patients, but fell short of banning the drugs.

In the UK, NICE (National Institute for Health and Clinical Excellence) recommended that no type of antidepressant should be used in the initial treatment of mild depression in adults or children, but for those deemed to be suffering moderate to severe depression, Prozac and Aropax should be favoured over other choices, based on comparisons of clinical data. Another UK body, the MHRA, advised that no SSRIs, except Prozac, be given to under-eighteens.

In Australia, nearly 200,000 PBS antidepressant prescriptions were written for people in the 16 to 20-year-old age group between 2003 and 2004. 14,421 were issued for children under the age of ten. In October 2004 the Therapeutic Goods Administration conducted its own study into the use of antidepressants in children and adolescents. Its paper reminded the medical community that *none* of the SSRIs (and indeed *no antidepressant*) is currently approved in Australia for the treatment of major depressive disorder in children and adolescents less than eighteen years. Two of the SSRIs, fluvoxamine and sertraline, are approved for children and adolescents with obsessive-compulsive disorder. The well-known risk of suicidal thoughts and the attempts at suicide that occur in adults during the early stages of antidepressant drug treatment had been shown to manifest in children and adolescents as well.

The TGA looked at the evidence from the USA, Australia and New Zealand, and formulated recommendations: SSRIs should only be used "within the context of comprehensive management of the patient", which is to say, you can't give an adolescent a prescription and send them on their way.

The chief medical officer of the TGA issued a statement in January 2005 indicating that if the growing antidepressant usage figures did not begin to moderate by mid-year he would refer the matter to a committee with the power to restrict the use of pharmaceuticals.

Elizabeth Wurtzel (herself not long out of her adolescent years at time of starting her book *Prozac Nation*) writes: "a little bit of energy is a dangerous thing in the hands of someone hell-bent on suicide, a very dangerous thing. My 'improved affect' [that is, applying for a job, paying back money, getting out of bed] did not sway me from my philosophical conviction that life sucks."

Ellie, at age eighteen, had six months of counselling for persistent sadness and non-coping symptoms following the break-up of the family home. She was not doing well ("If anything, I felt worse at these sessions") and the counsellor referred her to a doctor. She emerged after ten minutes with a prescription for mirtazapine (Avanza), and feels that she was left by the doctor to manage her confusion and unhappiness without any context except that the drugs would make her feel better. "I fell into this weird state of nothingness. I was in limbo, not happy, not sad, just a nothing person. And I had the worst nightmares. Really bad ones where I woke up screaming. Three times a week I'd wake up scared, then when I got back to sleep it was deep and heavy and felt like death." Ellie persisted for six months then stopped taking the drug.

She moved to another part of the state with her mother and enrolled in a course of study. A renewal of domestic stability, new friends and academic goals "made [her] feel like a real person again", an attitude that persisted until her mother left on a necessary and prolonged business trip which plunged her back into uncertainty and loneliness. She found her packet of Avanza and took a tablet, then after two particularly bad days where a series of small, otherwise manageable mishaps "did something to [her] head", Ellie crashed her car into a tree after taking a bend too quickly on a wet road. It is speculative to attribute her accident to a suicide attempt (she was shaken but not hurt), but the possibility has to be considered. Certainly her family rallied to make sure that she recovered in a cocoon of concerned attention. When I asked her what happened, she dismissed suicidal thoughts but admitted that the accident had brought its own benefits. Her car was a write-off but she now had friends who drove her to and from college, and a renewed sense that "people cared."

The drug given to eighteen-year-old Ellie, Avanza, is a non-SSRI antidepressant that is expressly not approved for use in children by the

American FDA. In Australia, the drug and others like it have been subjected to less scrutiny than the SSRIs and, says our TGA, "may be inefficacious and also associated with suicidality, as well as having other undesirable side effects such as the toxicity of the tricyclics in overdose".

Many hope the Therapeutic Goods Administration will be able to effect change through lobbying, but often the outcome amounts only to the inclusion of an extra paragraph in the patient information leaflet that accompanies the drug, hardly a neon sign warning of danger.

Why has it taken so long for us to hear about the increased risk of suicide in young people who take SSRIs? (Compare for instance the time line between approving and withdrawing Vioxx from sale, 1999–2004; SSRIs have been with us over a decade.)

The answer brings us back to the systemic problem at the heart of how we know what we know. Clinical trials are funded by pharmaceutical companies. Even our own TGA is funded by drug company money. Many of the clinical papers I've examined in my reading for this essay disclose that one or other of the authors owns stock in big pharma, or has received honoraria from various drug companies, and that expensive data from approved sources "were provided at no charge by [insert any drug company name]". There is no sin in using the service if it is offered, and indeed everything laudable in disclosing affiliations. The oversight, in my view, is in not recognising how interwoven big pharma is in the fabric of health delivery systems. Pull out the threads and the whole thing collapses. No money for research projects, no funding for trials, no conferences, fewer papers.

We have no routine blood tests or X-rays that will measure the subjective symptom we call "mood". But we do have simple measuring tools at our fingertips on the internet. Depression has been repackaged into soundbites and user-friendly quizzes on websites (with a handy reading age of fourteen years).

I took the online Goldberg Depression Quiz, first published in the

British Medical Journal in 1988 (and probably a bit outdated now since initiatives like *beyondblue*). Typing in my age and sex, and answering nine yes/no questions, I scored 7. "Only 8% of adults report as many or more depressive symptoms and 92% report fewer symptoms. The quiz cannot provide a professional diagnosis. However *you are reporting an unusually high number of depressive symptoms and it is possible you are depressed. We recommend you see a doctor.*" I took the test on 10 March 2005 and I'm trying to recall if I was having a blue or black day, or whether I was being deliberately wilful in faking a mood.

In another place I've written about my own struggle with anxiety and hypervigilance following a trauma in my adolescence. My nervous system is keenly alert to the jumpy, chaotic, jangly world of sudden stimuli. And what I've learnt is that anxiety is exhausting, and has its flipside — a sort of worn-out flatness which may look like (but I suspect is not) genuine depression. Early this year, in one of those depleted states I spoke to my doctor and filled in a K10 test, on which I also scored like a depressive. We are well acquainted, my GP and I, and on impulse I suggested it might be depression (I was weepy) and decided to trial Zoloft, to see if it made any difference. (Why not? I debated with myself, everyone else is taking it, it seems.)

However, Zoloft and I did not hit it off from day one. Even on half a 50mg tablet (my start-up dose), I was catapulted into a state of nervous anxiety. Sleep vanished. When I finally dozed I was woken by night terrors. Against all advice I stopped the drug after five days. Of course, I did it properly, tapering by increments and taking note of any unexpected reactions.

This may seem a hypocritical course of action in a pharmacist charged with keeping patients on track with their medications, and I relate it here for a number of reasons. Even when I was weeping on my doctor, I knew it was exhaustion; I knew it would heal itself with rest and distraction and comfort from people who cared. I also knew that I was asking for a short-cut to feeling better after a series of personal disappointments. Zoloft zealots (and there are many) extravagantly praise the drug's positive effects, and in a weak moment I wanted some of the action.

There is no confusion in my mind about encouraging a young woman like Angie to stay on her medication when she is far from home and vulnerable, while at the same time condoning my behaviour in jumping overboard at the first sign of upheaval. I've been a student of my own nervous system for long enough to know when I've put the wrong thing in my mouth.

We are, after all, the best arbiters of our own happiness. We know which way the wind is blowing (if we're in our right minds) and in all matters, particularly health, a little intelligence is our best defence against foolish mistakes. *Caveat emptor* also applies to prescription drugs.

Across counters in pharmacies all over the country, neat, labelled packets of pills meet their intended target, the ready and willing consumer. The transaction has a superficial resemblance to other commercial practices, but hidden from view are the suspension bridge-strength cables that lock the major participants into a tight embrace.

The small ritual of signing a legal document and paying a fee embodies the hopes of at least three competing groups: the physician (amelioration of symptoms), the drug company (bottom-line profit) and the patient.

It is not easy to summarise the hopes of the patient between brackets. Clearly, patients want to feel better. Not so clearly, they want to feel secure that the choice that has been made for them (drug A rather than drug B, or no drug at all) is a considered, unbiased decision based on sound medical judgment.

Things are changing, and so they should, given the Rand Corporation study of 1993 which revealed that more than half of surveyed US physicians consulted for less than three minutes with patients who claimed to be depressed before writing a prescription. I doubt that there are many practitioners today who believe that depression takes place in or emanates from a neurophysiological vacuum. Every right-thinking health professional frames the scientific message in a pastoral context: take this drug and seek counselling, join a support group, improve your diet, get some exercise.

In Australia the increase in numbers of scripts for antidepressants has been noted, and the need to pause and re-assess has been recognised. New National Prescribing Service guidelines have been issued which include six paragraphs on the option: "Consider psychological therapy as initial treatment in mild depression or as an adjunct to drug therapy in more severe depression." Our general practitioners are being "upskilled" through Commonwealth-funded initiatives like Better Outcomes in

Mental Health Care and the GP Care service, younger patients are being directed to computer-based interactive cognitive behaviour therapy programs, but we have stopped short of black-box warnings and strict guidelines on prescribing drugs for mild depression.

It is a truism of medical practice in this country that a prescription is proof that the patient is being taken seriously. The patient emerges from the consultation revivified by a medical diagnosis, which satisfies a deep need to be recognised as suffering (you are depressed), but veers well away from the much deeper fear the person brought with them and has barely dared to voice (you are mad).

In a small pharmacy where I sometimes work, I had three antidepressant conversations one after the other one autumn afternoon. Changes in the weather and season can bring out clusters of people with the same or similar prescriptions, and on this day there were three consecutive "Zoloft ladies". The first was a nurse who had taken herself off the drug after two years, lasted three months and was spiralling down into a bad place again. By her own diagnosis she was progressing from a unipolar into a bipolar disorder, and her question concerned titrating herself back up to the 150mg dose she'd been on at her worst. The second was an office worker who had tried a number of SSRIs before finding a measure of peace with Zoloft. Her question concerned the generic equivalent and the cost comparison since Zoloft attracted a surcharge on 1 April 2005. The third had stopped the drug after five years to give herself a break, and was coping – but in a different way from the way she coped while taking the drug. She'd forgotten how high the highs could get, and was consequently worried about the onset of lows. In light of all I'd read and thought about antidepressants I took particular notice of these conversations. They form, after all, a large part of my professional life in pharmacy. What was striking was the common assumption underlying each case, and my responses. Our starting point was an unstated acknowledgment that the drug cure was central to their individual depressions. What was at issue were the details. What dose? What price? What happens when I stop and want to start again? Our separate discussions (though valuable and pertinent) were further examples of piling up lesser things high enough to block out the view of the thing itself, the drug.

Later on the same day a drug company rep called in. She had driven a long way and had further to go before dark. This was new territory so she was ticking the essentials off her list: she asked about the local doctors, told me the names of her products and let me know whom she'd be detailing over the next few days.

Pharmacists have the ear of the public but they don't prescribe, so there is no mileage in pushing the message too hard. This young lady, who was clearly exhausted, said to me, with a nod to my years of experience of seeing company reps and our mutual desire to cut to the chase: "So what do you like, the presents or the information?" She unclipped her briefcase and drew out a clutch of pens. I broke out in a smile. A lone honest voice in the land of hard sell. No doubt she would rethink that encounter as she sped up the freeway and worry about the possible consequences, or maybe she'd be too tired to care. I certainly didn't. I put the pens in our pen drawer, already bulging with drug company giveaways, and filed the glossy brochure under its alphabetical letter.

Drug companies are important, and it is worth acknowledging that without them people like myself might have spent their working lives grinding roots in a mortar and pestle. The drug reps I've seen over many years are in the main proud of what they do, and are loyal to their companies. During training they absorb the company's values: innovative discoveries at great cost, margins which reflect their huge investment in research and development, the bringing to market of drugs that increase life expectancy and decrease days lost from work. These servants of big pharma are not privy to the shenanigans that go on at the top and I am not denigrating the work they do in bringing the messages into the field of action. (Nor am I criticising the GPs who receive the messages, or the pharmacists who fill the prescriptions and make their own profits from the transaction.)

Marcia Angell has proposed a prescription to heal the canker in big pharma. She notes that her recipe is idealistic, that achieving some of the changes is a "formidable" task, but in proposing an ideal she is giving the drug companies (and governments) something to aim for. She describes the canker by naming its traits. Many of the items on her hit-list have been alluded to in this essay. The over-involvement of drug companies in clinical research on their own products, their over-pervasive influence in educating doctors about their own products, their too-close alliance with the body that seeks to regulate them (the TGA in Australia's case), the misrepresentation of dollars they spend on R & D versus marketing, and the real lack of innovative new drugs, which is after all the moral justification for their continuance in the market. The last point relates to the proliferation of copy drugs (the so-called "me-too" drugs). Antidepressants have a few contenders in this category (Lexapro is one), but it applies particularly to the statins, the cholesterol-lowering drugs like Lipitor. When a market leader emerges and is doing well, the copycat drugs emerge fairly quickly. They are all variants on the original with little to distinguish one from the other (although the drug reps will labour the details of differentiation). Making copies by altering a few molecules is a lot cheaper than inventing a new drug from scratch.

Immediately one reads about me-too drugs, a host of comparisons come to mind: me-too books, me-too six-cylinder sports cars, me-too mixed alcoholic drinks. Big pharma is not the only player in town. The hostility I encountered from two Australian drug company spokesmen reflects the degree of protective allegiance they feel to their masters. It is also the defiance of someone caught in the act who shouts, "He's doing it too!"

The cure, according to Angell, is to disempower big pharma by strengthening the FDA (a worthy ambition for our own TGA). She also advocates an independent institute to oversee product testing. "Drug companies should no longer be permitted to control clinical testing of their own drugs." Her most strident call to arms is one that will resonate

with many observers in Australia: "Get big pharma out of medical education. We need an end to the fiction that big pharma provides medical
education. Drug companies are in business to sell drugs. Period."

I admired the small honesty afforded me by the exhausted drug rep
who couldn't be bothered going into her spiel when we both knew that
the purpose of her visit was to imprint a brand-name on my mind
through the wooing tactic of a handful of pens.

I suspect that Australians bought into depression (called misery-chic in the 1990s) about ten years after it hit the United States. It is not going to go away in a hurry and may even get worse.

How realistic is it to posit a "new" new order in which a modern GP could turn back the clock to a time when treatments were simpler, not drug-based, perhaps educational, supportive? A return, say, to traditional depression cures like borage flowers in wine, drunk *al fresco* with friends while wearing new clean clothes on a sunny day, after a good night's sleep and a bowel movement?

A prescription like this doesn't need a drug rep's endorsement or brand reminders. It does, however, require a major repositioning of ourselves as consumers. We may have to discard some ideas: that life equates to entertainment; that a bad day is somehow a bad movie for which we are entitled to a refund from the video hire shop (with the added satisfaction of complaining to the management). We may have to take responsibility for our own happiness. We may have to consider, like Nietzsche, that "the worst sickness of men has originated in the way they have combated their sickness. What seemed a cure has in the long run produced something worse than what it was supposed to overcome."

But what about a depressed twenty-something girl who self-harms, or the surly boy in the next street? Of what use is a recipe like the one above to someone who cannot take the reins of their lives? Do we deny them the chemical equivalent of a helping hand when the trees are rushing past and their carriage is headed for a cliff? I think not. I think we allow for the great blessing of living in a country where we can exercise free will; and make good use of our intelligence to find the right help at the right moment. The drugs may be uniform in dose and presentation; we are not.

Did all the saved string change the course of the economic depression of 1930s? Hardly, but it made a lot of people feel that they had a small part to play in controlling what threatened to overwhelm their lives.

*

Angie is now settled in New York, still taking her Zoloft because she's worried that she'd be volatile without it, and conscious that she doesn't have her home-based support network to pick her up if she falls. "But being here and having time to myself has made me really question how much my moods and behaviour depend on chemistry alone. I thought about that idea that depression just allows people a bit of natural downtime and I think I agree. I think my body has been aching for this break for a very long time and my brain is finally ready to move into new habits."

Back at the beginning of my talk with Angie, she said, "I've read Foucault. But that's my choice — taking Zoloft makes me feel better."

I had to ask a friend to interpret this remark for me. "Antidepressants could be seen as promoting a certain level of happiness *as an acceptable norm*," he wrote. "In other words, in the act of taking an antidepressant, you are giving in to society and social mores. A comment like 'I've read Foucault and I take Zoloft' is akin to saying 'Yes, I wear Nike shoes, and yes, I've read *No Logo*.'"

I suspect it is easier for the generation to which Angie belongs to sustain these simultaneous contradictions. From where I stand in the sequence of generations, I know (and brood over) the fact that big pharma is still shaping the social as well as the medical landscape when I hear Bette Midler, now fifty-nine, making jokes about "the Lipitor years".

I finished the first draft of this essay in Katoomba in the Blue Mountains west of Sydney. Hiking up the main street one afternoon I stopped to look at leaflets pinned to a noticeboard. A band was playing on Saturday night. *Fluoxetine*. In an hallucinatory few seconds I thought my obsessive reading about depression had painted the whole world in SSRI colours. I had another look. *Fluoxetine*: the name of a band which promised a night of Alter-Alternative Hard Rock & Jazzy Latiny Funk, and the chemical name of Prozac, science's gift (via Eli Lilly and Company) to the late twentieth century.

ABBREVIATIONS

ABS   Australian Bureau of Statistics
ADD   Attention Deficit Disorder
ADHD   Attention Deficit Hyperactivity Disorder
ADRAC   Adverse Drug Reactions Advisory Committee
APMA   Australian Pharmaceutical Manufacturers Association
BMJ   British Medical Journal
CBT   Cognitive Behaviour Therapy
COX-2   Cyclooxygenase-2 inhibitor, stated to selectively inhibit an enzyme in the inflammation pathway (now known to also inhibit an enzyme in the blood-clotting pathway)
DTC   Direct to Customer (advertising)
FDA   Food and Drug Administration (USA)
GP   General practitioner
IMS   Intercontinental Marketing Services
MHRA   Medicines and Healthcare Products Regulatory Authority (UK)
MJA   Medical Journal of Australia
NaSSA   (sometimes NASSA) Noradrenergic and specific serotonergic antidepressant
NPS   National Prescribing Service
OCD   Obsessive-compulsive disorder
PBS   Pharmaceutical Benefits Scheme
R & D   Research & development
SNRI   Serotonin noradrenergic reuptake inhibitor
SSRI   Selective serotonin reuptake inhibitor
TCA   Tricyclic antidepressant
TGA   Therapeutic Goods Australia
WHO   World Health Organization

SOURCES

2   "postmodern girl's dilemma": private email correspondence with "Angie" after our first meeting.

3   All statistics in this essay are derived from the following sources (viewed between January and April 2005) unless otherwise stated: PBS, IMS Health Inc, ABS, MJA, TGA www.tga.gov.au, BMJ.

4   William Styron. *Darkness Visible: A Memoir of Madness*, Random House, New York, 1990.

5   Ray Moynihan & Alan Cassels, *Selling Sickness: How Drug Companies Are Turning Us All into Patients*, Allen & Unwin, Sydney, 2005. See also *British Medical Journal*, 324, 2002, pp. 886–891.

6   "change fatigue" and personal resilience: these issues are complex, and outside the scope of this essay. I direct the reader to Hugh Mackay's 2005 Manning Clark Lecture, Social Disengagement: A Breeding Ground for Fundamentalism, 3 March 2005, www.abc.net.au/rn/bigidea/stories/s1323906.htm, and Richard Eckersley's *Well and Good: How We Feel and Why It Matters*, Text Publishing, Melbourne, 2004.

9   Elizabeth Wurtzel. *Prozac Nation: Young and Depressed in America*. Houghton Mifflin, Boston, 1994. I have quoted extensively from Wurtzel's book for all the reasons given by the *New York Times* in its original review: "Wrenching and comical, self-indulgent and self-aware, *Prozac Nation* possesses the raw candor of Joan Didion's essays, the irritating emotional exhibitionism of Sylvia Plath's *The Bell Jar*, and the wry, dark humour of a Bob Dylan song."

9   Hagen, Watson and Andrews: www.abc.net.au/rn/science/mind/stories/s1261369.htm. Taken from the transcript of *All in the Mind*, 15 January 2005, "The Evolution of Depression – Does it Have a Role?" Links and references are provided at the end of the transcript.

10   Rita Carter. *Mapping the Mind*, University of California Press, Berkeley, 1998, p. 102 in the 1999 paperback edition.

11   "entirely malleable": Carter, p. 6.

12   Kelsey Hegarty, "Management of Mild Depression in General Practice: Is Self-Help the Solution?" *Australian Prescriber*, Vol. 28, No. 1, February 2005, p. 10.

13   "feeling 'weird'": interview with patient "B" conducted by author.

15   "drug doctors and talk doctors": Sean Kelly, "Prozac Wars", University of Sydney, History IV thesis, 2001, available from the thesis library at the University of Sydney. I am indebted to Sean for his correspondence and for guiding me through theories of culture and identity. Any misunderstandings are mine.

16   "Tryptanol took off like a rocket": Carl Elliott, "American Bioscience Meets the American Dream", *The American Prospect*, Vol. 14, No. 6, 1 June 2003.

18   Marcia Angell, *The Truth about Drug Companies: How They Deceive Us and What To Do about It*, Random House, New York, 2004, p. 41.

20   1988 study: Roughead E.E., Harvey K.J., Gilbert A.L., "Commercial detailing techniques used by pharmaceutical representatives to influence prescribing", *Aust NZ Journal of Medicine*, 28, 1998, pp. 306–310.

20   388 reports: *Australian Adverse Drug Reactions Bulletin*, Vol. 13, No. 4, November 1994.

21   "clinical trials of Prozac": Ann Blake Tracy, *Prozac: Panacea or Pandora?*, Cassia Publications, Utah, 2004.

22   Angell, p. 112.

22–3   "Rofecoxib: a case in point", *NPS News*, No. 37, December 2004.

33   "papers on ... neuropsychiatry and women's issues": The Jean Hailes Foundation is a good starting point. www.jeanhailes.org.au.

34   "Older doctors": "Older doctors suffer the shock of the new", *Sydney Morning Herald*, 16 February 2005.

35   John J. Ratey and Catherine Johnson, *Shadow Syndromes: Recognizing and Coping with Hidden Psychological Disorders That Can Influence Your Behaviour & Silently Determine the Course of Your Life*, Pantheon, New York, 1997.

35   *Seinfeld* episode, "The Suicide", 1992.

41   "radical materialist ideology": Associate Professor Leon Petchovsky, quoted in *Complementary Medicine* magazine, Jan/Feb 2005, Institute of Australasian Psychiatrists' conference, November 2004.

44   "as big as a coconut": Carter, p. 15.

45–6   2002 study: Angell, p. 113.

46   "a paper from Massachusetts General Hospital": Dr Jerrold Rosenbaum, Chief of Psychiatry, Massachusetts General Hospital, Boston, quoted in www.depressionissues.com/ms/news/519999/main.html. Viewed on 21/2/2005.

48   "fighting depression on two fronts": "The Placebo Effect", *The Health Report*, ABC Radio National, 7 March 2005, Dr Norman Swan in conversation with Helen Mayberg, Professor of Psychiatry and Neurology, Emory University, Atlanta, Georgia.

48–9   R.F.W. Moulds, "Expensive new drugs – do we really need them?", *Australian Prescriber*, Vol. 27, No. 6, December 2004, p. 136.

51   "Books on Prescription": Wendy Champagne, "A Cheerful Note on Depression", *Sydney Morning Herald*, 3 March 2005.

61   "We have no routine blood tests": There is the rarely used dexamethasone suppression test (DST), performed by giving 1mg of dexamethasone at 11 p.m. and measuring serum cortisol the next day at 4 p.m. and 11 p.m. Fifty per cent of melancholics fail to suppress cortisol, but there is no current consensus on the sensitivity or specificity of the findings.

62   "trauma in my adolescence": Gail Bell, SHOT: *A Personal Response to Guns and Trauma*, Picador, Sydney, 2003.

62   "K10 test": Kessler Psychological Distress Scale, used to assess a patient's condition and change over time. One of the outcome tools recommended for use by Australian GPs. It is in the public domain and can be accessed at www.crufad.org.

64   "for less than three minutes": Wurtzel, p. 338.

64   "New NPS guidelines": National Prescribing Service, Prescribing Practice Review (PPR27) for General Practice, *Managing Depression*, August 2004.

Elizabeth Evatt & Richard Chisholm

John Hirst's essay, though flawed by errors and by ill-concealed bias, raises some important issues about family law. There are three main components of Hirst's essay: the invective, the case summaries and the proposals for law reform.

By invective, the sort of thing we have in mind is the use of "kangaroo court", references to judges not caring about injustice, the court abusing children, and – most memorably – the suggestion that judges are like Nazis (because they followed the High Court's ruling about the approach to be taken in child abuse cases – more of this later). While such comments may grab headline attention, they do little to advance debate on serious issues.

The second component is the case summaries, mainly the stories of three fathers, called in the essay Paul Walton, Graham Sweetland and Julian Aston. These histories form a considerable part of the basis for the discussion and proposals, so they need consideration.

Graham Sweetland

Graham Sweetland failed in his attempt to gain residence of a baby boy: the outcome of the case was that he had contact every second weekend and half school holidays. John Hirst seems to agree with Graham's view that the Family Court will "treat him for a time as a pariah" and with his bitterness over the money he spent and "what happened to his reputation". He refers to "the static of false allegations" and asks, "Who knows how much notice the court takes of allegations?" Certainly Hirst's readers don't, because we do not know what allegations were made at the trial, or whose evidence the Court accepted, or about either party's ability to care for the child. It is not clear whether Hirst even asked Graham to see a copy of the judgment.

The chapter ends with Hirst saying how much better it will all be when the adversary system is replaced by the inquisitorial method, referring with approval to the Family Court's Children's Cases Project. We agree that these initiatives are promising. But even if they succeed in eliminating irrelevant material and streamlining the proceedings, the Court (or any decision-making body) will still have to deal with allegations relevant to children's safety and wellbeing in the care of those competing to have the children live with them.

Paul Walton

After separation, Paul had an "argument" with one of his two daughters, after which his contact tailed off. Paul's wife accused him of being "verbally abusive and physically intimidating"; and the children themselves wrote to say, "You are not our Dad and we don't want anything to do with you." After attempts to re-establish contact with the children Paul decided not to make an application to the courts. The only involvement of the Family Court is at the end when a counsellor helps the parties resolve a question about supplying school reports to Paul (who was "highly complimentary" about the Court's counsellor).

Hirst seems to accept Paul's view that this is an example of the "Parent Alienation Syndrome". The reader cannot possibly know whether to agree, since we only have Paul's side of the story, and much is omitted. We are told something about Paul's feelings of impotence and distress at having the children "stolen" from him. But we never learn why, if Paul was the "primary parent", the parties agreed that the children would live mostly with their mother. We are not told the nature of the "argument" that led to the visits tailing off. We never learn how Paul's bipolar disorder affected his behaviour, or what was the "disturbing history about the difficulties over the years relevant to contact" that the wife's solicitor wrote about.

Hirst seems content to rely on what others told Paul about the Family Court. For example, Paul's doctor told him that medical records could be used selectively against him, and that legal aid would not assist. In fact, it is not possible for one side to put before the Court only restricted parts of medical reports: the Court would want to see the whole of each relevant report. As for legal aid, there seems no reason to think that if Paul passed the needs test he would not have got legal aid for a contact application, and in a case like this there would almost certainly be a separate legal representative for the children.

There are many cases where parents give up in the face of opposition to contact, and we could learn a lot from them and perhaps find ways of helping to maintain positive relationships between the parents themselves and the parents and their children. Unfortunately, Hirst's account is too partisan to be a useful contribution on this subject. He can only see Paul's point of view: not that of the wife, not that of the children.

The denigration of the Court becomes farcical at the end of this chapter, where Hirst says that this is "a standard Family Court procedure: the excluded parent indicates that they will abandon attempts to see the child in return for receiving news of them." There is of course no such procedure. The court does not choose the terms on which parties negotiate, or the outcome of the negotiations. Here, the Court did the only thing it was asked, namely to help the parties resolve a question about school reports, the only issue they chose to raise. Paul's story does not in any way support Hirst's denigration of the Family Court or his proposals for law reform.

Julian Aston

Julian Aston's story is a desperate saga involving a mother who persistently made false allegations of sexual abuse, avoided court orders and poisoned the child against the father over a six-year period of investigations and hearings by a range of courts and child welfare authorities. The courts consistently accepted the truth of the father's evidence, and consistently disbelieved the mother, and found that the father had not abused the child and that there was no risk of abuse. Nevertheless, at the end of it all the father had lost contact with the daughter, and can only hope she seeks him out in years to come. It must have been a devastating and destructive experience for both father and daughter: a tragic outcome, and a horrible process.

Hirst's conclusion is that the Family Court is "a child abuser". A more accepted term for Hirst's point is "systems abuse", on which there is a large international literature. It is well known that tragically in some situations the interventions of child protection agencies, and various courts, can themselves make things worse for the child.

Identifying occurrences of systems abuse is important, and this case might well merit a thorough examination. Identifying the problem, of course, is easier than solving it. Nobody would say that all child abuse allegations should be disregarded; but as soon as one starts to investigate, there is the potential for the investigative processes to have an adverse impact. Hirst, with the benefit of hindsight, is critical of a number of decisions made in the course of this saga. He may be right. But his account underplays some of the difficulties.

For example, he seems to argue that after the first court finding favouring the father, all further allegations should have been dismissed "as coming from a totally unreliable source". He is referring here to the mother. But it seems from his account that the child herself was making the allegations. By the end of the dreadful period, it had become apparent that there was no truth in them; but this may not have been so obvious in the earlier stages. Hirst seems to argue that any fresh allegation of sexual assault by the young child should have been disregarded, and not investigated at all. But that conclusion could only be responsibly reached by carefully considering the evidence that was available at the time.

Penalising breach of contact orders

Hirst correctly identifies an imbalance between enforcing child support and contact: those seeking to enforce child-support orders (mainly mothers) have the benefit of a public agency, while those seeking to enforce contact orders (mainly fathers) have to bring proceedings themselves. As legal aid is often not available for these cases, bringing numerous applications to deal with successive incidents can easily run up legal bills that the fathers cannot meet, and indeed may lead them to give up in despair, as it is difficult to succeed in these proceedings without legal representation. Courts cannot assist here: they can only adjudicate on applications, in this case applications by the contact parent to penalise the other parent for breach of the order. There may well be a need to allocate additional resources for the specific task of dealing with problems of non-compliance constructively at an early stage, treating the implementation of the Court's orders as requiring a public response, rather than being a burden on the other parent.

In other respects, however, the discussion is less helpful. The argument seems to be that the Family Court should enforce its orders more vigorously. Hirst refers to the Court's "poor record", says the Court has not been concerned about upholding its authority, says that its orders are "a joke", and so on. But despite the vehemence of these comments, it is difficult to identify just what Hirst proposes. He notes, without apparently disagreeing, that none of the various bodies that have conducted inquiries into the problem favoured "sharp punitive methods, that is, to lock up a few offenders in the hope that the rest would fall into line".

Part of the difficulty may be that Hirst seems to believe, wrongly, that the courts treat the child's best interests as paramount in these cases; in fact, the well-known "paramount consideration" principle has never applied to proceedings for penalties.[1] The law requires the Court to weigh up in each case the often-competing considerations of upholding the court's authority (by penalising breaches) and having regard to the child's interests. If Hirst concedes that some such balancing process is appropriate, then his criticism would require him to show that the Court has got the balance wrong in particular cases, a task that would require a more thorough analysis than could be attempted in an essay of this kind.

Hirst's colourfully expressed conclusion, that the Court does not *care* about maintaining the relationship between fathers and children, no doubt reflects the views of the men he spoke to, who were understandably frustrated at being separated from their children notwithstanding court orders for contact. But we think it is mistaken, because it underestimates the difficulties of fostering these relationships in the midst of family conflict, difficulties which have been the reason why the series of reviews and inquiries Hirst refers to have not led to recommendations, or legislation, creating a more punitive system.

There are, perhaps, three main problems. The first is that in many cases the fathers have been unable to establish that there has been a breach (perhaps a Contact Compliance Service would ease this problem). The second is that in some situations the penalty may cause the child to suffer: financial penalties may have an adverse impact on a low-income household, and imprisoning the mother might harm the child, especially if there are no other suitable people to care for the child while the mother is in prison. There is no doubt room for argument about how these factors should be balanced in each case: but to reach a conclusion, we would need to know all the facts.

The third problem is perhaps the most important of all. A breakdown in the children's relationship with the father in these cases is a tragic outcome for the children, as well as deeply distressing for the fathers. But because of the complex dynamics of the relationships, penalties, even if initially successful in having the child physically transferred to the father for contact, may escalate the level of conflict and bitterness, and bring about a situation which damages, rather than improves, the father–child relationship, to the detriment of both. It is naive to suggest that taking a tougher line on defaulting mothers will necessarily have the desired result, as Hirst appears to do when he says that by not pressuring a mother who is unco-operative about contact, the Court "has left large numbers of children without an effective father".

Hirst does not identify precisely what he would like the law to say, but it seems that he would want the Court to emphasise punishment of those who breach orders, if necessary at the expense of the children. But it is by no means clear that this approach would usually lead to better outcomes, either for the fathers or the children. The Court cannot transform people who are unreasonable and vindictive into responsible and reasonable adults. Its power to punish is a blunt weapon, which could do as much or more damage than it cures. Any chance there may have been of gradually building working relationships between the parents may well be shattered, and children caught up in the parental conflict may suffer great distress. Often a "least worst" solution is all that can be offered.

Obstructing contact ordered by the Court without a reasonable excuse is wrong, and it is easy to say that punishment is warranted. But preserving and enhancing a positive relationship between the father and the child in these situations can be acutely difficult, and often requires a far more subtle and understanding response. Enforcing contact in a situation where the parent or children suffer severe stress and anxiety is of little benefit to anyone. That is why the effort is made, through counselling, to help the parties to deal with each other civilly at the earliest possible opportunity, and to work out a solution to meet their needs. The best way to ensure effective involvement of both parents in the ongoing care of their children is to foster a working relationship between those parents (excluding cases where violence or other danger is involved).

When Hirst says it would be better for the Court to "work for a settlement which as far as possible kept both parents involved in the lives of their children", he is echoing the Act, which gives parents the obligation to agree about the future parenting of their children after separation. The Act aims to encourage parents to take responsibility for parenting arrangements, to use the legal system as a last resort and to regard the best interests of their children as the paramount consideration. That is why counselling services are provided as part of the family law system.

One feature of the law, particularly in the recent reforms to which Hirst refers, is to ensure that the contact orders themselves can be re-examined. Perhaps there has developed an arbitrary formula of alternate weekends and half the holidays, and it can be very helpful to explore alternatives, especially if the parents and those advising them are able to think creatively about an arrangement that will help each parent in their future parenting roles. We are increasingly realising that in some situations, especially with skilled and sensitive assistance, the children themselves can contribute to finding a solution. The Court knows that it is far better for a solution to be worked out by the parties than to be dictated by a court order prescribing the times, places and dates for delivery and collection of children. Such orders impose a rigid legal framework on the pattern of family life, remote from the realities of unexpected change, and adjusted timetables which are the common experience of us all. Many responsible parents make flexible arrangements for sharing the future care of their children, arrangements which suit their particular needs and which can be varied readily as the situation changes.

Child sexual abuse

Another concern of Hirst is the denial or restriction of contact by a parent against whom allegations of sexual abuse have been made. He argues that the Family Court should make a definitive finding one way or the other about the allegations of abuse – the person accused must be judged guilty or innocent.

Even if this were a good idea, the Family Court could not do it. Its present approach is required by law: the *Family Law Act*, as interpreted by the High Court in the M *and* M case, which he discusses. If there is to be a change, it is necessary for parliament to amend the Act.

Should there be a change? Opinions will no doubt differ, and the High Court ruling has its critics. But we think Hirst underestimates the difficulties with his proposal. The High Court pointed out that there will be very many cases where the court *cannot* confidently make a finding that sexual abuse has taken place. "*And there are strong practical family reasons why the court should refrain from making a positive finding that sexual abuse has taken place unless it is impelled by the particular circumstances to do so.*" The Court's task, it held, is to determine the magnitude of the risk: "the test is best expressed by saying that a court will not grant custody or contact to a parent if that custody or contact would expose the child to an unacceptable risk of sexual abuse." The Family Court is bound by this High Court decision.

In these distressing cases the evidence is often ambiguous, the allegations strongly denied, and the experts divided or uncertain, both about whether the abuse has occurred and about what should be done (not all cases are like that of Julian Aston). In these proceedings, the Court is usually assisted by hearing from the child's representative and independent experts such as child psychiatrists. In such cases judges sometimes conclude that the protection of the child against risk of abuse must prevail over the distress to the person against whom the allegations are made. Would Hirst want the courts to ignore such a risk in the many cases where the evidence does not permit a firm finding that abuse has taken place?

The distress of a father whose contact is restricted or denied in these circumstances is understandable, even tragic. But we do not think that this problem can be resolved by requiring the Court to order contact where it is satisfied that doing so would expose the child to an unacceptable risk of abuse. Such an adult-centred approach would displace proper concern for the child.

There is no space to deal with the passage at the end of this chapter, in which Hirst offers a "summary" of the Family Court's approach. We simply note that this summary misrepresents the situation, and fails to address the crucial issue, namely what action the Court should take when the evidence leads to the conclusion that there is an unacceptable risk of abuse.

Other proposals

Another of Hirst's proposals is that the law should recognise the legal right of a parent to see his or her children, unless likely to do them harm. In this, as in some other respects, he takes an adult-centred approach, whereas the *Family Law Act* is child-centred. It recognises not the rights of parents, but their shared duties and responsibilities, including the obligation to agree about future parenting. The Act also recognises the right of children to know and be cared for by both parents, and to have contact with both parents, unless this would be contrary to their best interests. The Family Court is required to consider the individual feelings, thoughts and wishes of the children, the nature of their relationship with each parent, and other factors, in determining their best interests. We cannot share Hirst's desire to turn away from these matters and enforce a parental right regardless of the child's best interests, excepting only the situation of likely harm.

Hirst would also like the law to be changed to relieve a parent of his child-support payments if court-ordered contact is denied. But this would lead to two wrongs instead of one: denial of contact ordered by the Court is wrong, and so is failure to pay child support. Withholding child support is not a valid means of enforcing contact, since children must still be fed, clothed and sheltered.

Another of Hirst's proposals is that refusal of contact ordered by the Court should result in the transfer of custodial care, if the other parent is *adequate to the task*, regardless of the child's wishes or feelings. We doubt that this formula would be likely to promote either successful contact, or stability and security in relationships, which children of broken relationships deserve. In this as in some other recommendations, Hirst argues for an adult-centred rather than a child-centred approach to family law.

Back to absolutism?

The key underlying theme of Hirst's approach is that the "best interests of the child" principle should be replaced by a set of absolutist rules, which must be applied *even if the Court believes the application of such rules would not be in the best interests of the child*. For our part, we are not persuaded that Australia should abandon the principle that the best interests of children should be determined on a case-by-case basis. Children, who are too often the silent witnesses to the destructive behaviour of their parents, deserve better than a change that would take us back to the nineteenth century, and would, incidentally, be difficult to reconcile with Australia's obligations under the international Convention on the Rights of the Child.

Elizabeth Evatt & Richard Chisholm

1 Section 70NJ; compare s 65E, applying the "paramount consideration" principle to parenting orders (residence, contact, etc).

Correspondence

Peter Ryan

Nobody expected John Hirst's *"Kangaroo Court"* to tell a sunny story. The roots of the Australian Family Court feed so deep in swamps of human malignity and spite, in conjugal hate and juvenile pain that many of its fruits are bound to be poisonous. The Family Court is said to be the source of more complaints made by citizens to members of parliament than any other subject.

From Hirst's careful evidence I learned that this court drives litigants to suicide, does not enforce its own judgments, runs a poison-pen service, acts with heavy prejudice against male litigants (husbands), has allowed the proliferation of lawyers with their crippling bills of costs, inspires escalating perjuries, is a gross abuser of human rights and "is itself a child abuser". It is a failing institution which embodies the core moral contradictions of our age.

Whew!

Hirst treats the history of the Family Court as a product largely of Alastair Nicholson, its chief justice of some sixteen years, now lately retired. Many have seen him in the same light as Hirst – as a judicial practitioner of wrong-headed self-righteousness – though it is rare for him to draw criticism from feminists. The former Chief Justice maintained his own steady course, undeflected by the cries of pain and dismay, and in the face even of legislative attempts to point Australia's divorce law in a less destructive direction.

Hirst's main objective did not require him to provide any more personal information about His Honour than the *Quarterly Essay* sets out. Yet many a reader may feel curious about what manner of man presided over the court which bulldozed such changes into the Australian landscape of marriage and family. Nicholson has forthrightly proclaimed his position, and resolutely defended it, not only from the bench, but also in the public forum. By many observers over the past sixteen years, he was seen as a rubicund and imperturbable judicial Mr Toad, motoring along with his exhaust on fire, as he waved gaily to the frantic crowds trying to warn him of his peril.

In fact, Alastair Nicholson enjoyed an unusual breadth of judicial experience, for he was for some six years a judge of the Supreme Court of Victoria, and held office also as a judge of the Federal Court. From 1987 to 1992 he was (presumably in a peacetime, part-time capacity) Judge Advocate General of the Australian Defence Force. Though he has left his Family Court behind, it seems unlikely that we will cease to hear the strong and undoubtedly sincere opinions of Alastair Nicholson.

Hirst's story of the Family Court leaves its appalled reader suspended between tears and rage: the shattered lives, the ruined reputations, the bankruptcies that follow the legal bills, the enduring juvenile doubt and pain – surely all these might be made the stuff of drama, when they come to their next telling?

Not a sociologist, not a lawyer, not a psychologist, not a social worker, John Hirst is a *historian*, whom decency and conscience persuaded to make this long detour from his accustomed work. But the training and the habits of a historian have strengthened his arm. His ugly tale emerges from facts carefully assembled and tested; the links in his chain of logic are well-welded and firm; his language is shiningly lucid. (I found not one sentence that needed two readings to extract a meaning.) Although his censure is sharp, his telling is always civil and calm.

Hirst has not been one to waste time on the futile academic sterilities of "history wars" and the like. He gets on with it, and shows that historians, after all, can actually be useful. This scorching *Quarterly Essay* furnishes a model for undergraduates everywhere – how the job should be done. Is it too much to hope that some established historians may read this, and learn something?

Peter Ryan

Alastair Nicholson

It is not my intention to reply in detail to the polemic written by John Hirst on the Family Court of Australia. It is so riddled with factual inaccuracies, misunderstandings of the law and the Australian court system, and so affected by actual bias and prejudice, that it is not worthy of a detailed reply to the whole of it.

It is also a debate upon grounds chosen by himself, in relation to which he appears to have made little attempt to check the accuracy of his assertions. I am quite happy to let my record as Chief Justice of the Family Court of Australia speak for itself without seeking to defend it from an attack such as this.

I do however propose to take up several matters that he raised which are of public interest and have a particular bearing on the Court's handling of issues that affect children.

The enforcement of contact orders

I think it important to discuss the enforcement of contact orders, if only to clarify and highlight some of the difficulties that do arise in the enforcement of contact orders, not only in this country but in all countries where a family jurisdiction exists, difficulties which have largely escaped Hirst.

Hirst asserts that the "disobeying of a court order is known as a contempt of court and is the offence that threatens the foundations of our society. We are governed by the rule of law and once courts have settled the law, it has to be obeyed by governments and citizens alike. To ensure that these orders are obeyed, courts have large, discretionary powers to fine and imprison those who defy them. Though it was to be a court of a new sort, the Family Court has been equipped with these powers."

This passage confuses two concepts, namely the role of courts in stating the law and their role in making orders. It also elevates court orders to a position that they have never occupied by suggesting that a breach of them threatens the foundations of our society. Many court orders, including most Family Court orders, are made by consent in terms drafted by the parties or their lawyers. Very often they contain unenforceable sections or their application covers situations that the parties never envisaged. In many cases circumstances have radically changed between the time of the making of the order and its proposed enforcement. To ascribe to them the force and status that Hirst seeks to do is misleading and wrong.

The fact is that the courts have and must have powers to enforce their orders. However this has always been a discretionary power that the court is not obliged to enforce if it considers that the particular circumstances do not require it. It also has a further discretion as to the type of enforcement or sanction, if any, that will be applied.

The Family Court, like all other courts, routinely does make orders for enforcement of orders. For example, orders for the payment of money, the transfer of property or directing that a child reside with a particular person are frequently made and where necessary enforced, usually without difficulty. Similarly, injunctions restraining a person from doing a certain act or more rarely requiring that something positive be done are frequently made and enforced. The situation in these cases is not very different from other civil courts. Like all other civil courts the Court does not of its own initiative enforce orders and enforcement only occurs at the instance of the person seeking to enforce the order.

The position of contact orders is somewhat different. Of course most people do comply with these orders and the more sensible agree to *de facto* modifications as time goes by to suit changing circumstances. The Court when called upon to do so enforces these orders also, but often that process is not as simple as Hirst attempts to portray.

An ordinary court order made by a civil court such as a Supreme Court usually arises out of a finding of a court as to the commission of a wrongful act by the defendant which the order seeks to redress. It is normally directed against a person who has been directly involved in the commission of the wrongful act or who has received property as a result of it. Often the order is made by default, but it may also follow the court having made a final adjudication as to the dispute, which is embodied in the order.

By contrast, a Family Court order for contact is not the result of the commission of a civil wrong. The parents of the child or children concerned have simply separated, and where they are unable to agree the Court is called upon to adjudicate as to the parent with whom the child should reside (if that is in dispute) and more commonly the amount and nature of the contact that should take place between the non-resident parent and the child. Before the Court is called upon to make that decision, there will have been an exhaustive attempt to mediate the dispute, which usually results in the making of consent orders.

A very distinctive feature of contact orders is that their primary effect is upon a person who is not only not party to the dispute, but has no voice in its resolution, namely the child (or children) concerned.

The orders, as Hirst concedes, are intended to operate over a lengthy period. This in itself gives rise to particular problems. Even if the initial arrangement between the parents is satisfactory to themselves and the child, other factors may quickly intervene such as re-partnering by one or both parents, often to partners who have their own children, and geographical and employment changes. The needs and requirements of children change as they grow older and circumstances change and these are often not envisaged by the order.

Even in the absence of such factors, it must be remembered that the contact order by its very nature imposes very significant obligations, not only upon the resident parent but upon the child. By contrast, no obligation whatever is imposed upon the non-resident parent. They can choose to avail themselves of the order or not as they see fit. They are free to move away, even to another country, and they can arrive to exercise their rights of contact when it suits them. There is usually no obligation upon them even to be punctual.

The extent of interference with the lifestyle of the resident parent is not often appreciated. Effectively they are required to remain in the one place and to produce the child when required by the order. Further, they must do this *regardless of the wishes of the child.*

That approach may be defensible in relation to very young children, but as children become older they very often develop strong views as to whether they wish contact to proceed or not. They may have good reason for this. There may be difficult relationships with the non-resident parent's new partner or siblings. They may have developed interests and activities that are seriously disrupted by the effect of the contact order. They may develop a very difficult relationship with the non-resident parent. The non-resident parent may be using contact entitlements as a means of controlling or punishing the resident parent. In worst-case scenarios, the non-resident parent may be physically, sexually or psychologically abusing one or more of the children.

It follows that the automatic enforcement of orders of this nature, as envisaged by Hirst, would be potentially disastrous. There are many instances where the making of the enforcement application highlights the unsuitability of the original order and the need to change it. Enforcement applications are frequently made for purely tactical reasons or with the intention to harass the other partner and put them to expense.

None of this means that contact orders need not be enforced in appropriate cases, but it does mean that the sort of simplistic approach advocated by Hirst concerning the enforcement of court orders is quite inappropriate. The child may be endangered by the enforcement of the orders, and the imprisonment or other punishment of the resident parent may not only be unjust but entirely counter-productive to the preservation of the relationship between the child and the non-resident parent.

The issue of enforcement of this type of order must be approached in the sensitive manner that I believe the Court has done.

In his essay, Hirst is highly critical of the Court for finding that as a matter of law, the right to contact is one of the child and not of the parent. That happens to represent the law as stated in the *Family Law Act*, but the reality is that he is tilting at a straw man in any case. The overall approach of the Court from its inception has favoured the preservation of contact with both parents and it is only in the rarest of cases that an order refusing contact is made. Indeed I think that a respectable argument could be mounted that the Court has been over-zealous in requiring contact, particularly in cases where there are serious allegations of violence or child abuse.

Hirst also suggests that despite the government's legislation providing for a three-stage enforcement regime, the Court somehow refused to comply with it. If he had done his homework, which he failed to do in so many areas, he would have found that the Court welcomed this legislation but complained bitterly to government that it had introduced this legislation but had failed to fund the organisations designated to provide services under it. It seems that only now has the government belatedly recognised this problem in the context of the 2005 Budget. Following the introduction of this legislation, I received many complaints from judges and had the experience myself of being unable to find any organisation able or willing to provide the services envisaged by it, simply because they had not been funded by the government to do so.

The one area that does cause me concern in relation to enforcement is the matter of how to deal with cases where there is a persistent and unjustified defiance of court orders for contact. These cases are very few but are troublesome. As Hirst correctly points out, the responsibility for bringing enforcement proceedings lies with the person seeking to enforce the order. Given the legal aid policies of this and previous governments, this can impose an impossible financial burden upon some people. Hirst is critical of the Court for requiring strict proof of breach of orders, but in this regard it is simply following the practice of other courts and in my view rightly so, given that the penalties for breach can include imprisonment. However it does mean that when people attempt to enforce orders without legal advice, there are often technical deficiencies in their applications.

The Court has been aware of this problem for some time, as is evidenced by the fact that in its 1991 submissions to the McKiernan Committee it urged that the Director of Public Prosecutions or some other Commonwealth agency accept responsibility for the enforcement of persistent breach of court orders. Similar suggestions have been made since, without result. As I see it, this is the only solution to this problem. It would be contrary to the principles of independence of courts for it to act as a prosecutor, and it therefore seems that this represents the only real alternative, other than a significant relaxation of legal aid guidelines.

Allegations of child sexual abuse

A further area that is worthy of comment is the issue of handling allegations of child sexual abuse. Hirst demonstrates a considerable ignorance of the law and practice in this area and the effect of the decided cases. Much of his criticism of the Family Court in this area relates to the decision of the High Court of Australia in M *and* M, for which the Family Court bears no responsibility and the principles of which bind its decisions in this area. He suggests that the proper test should be that the Court should be satisfied that abuse has occurred before taking it into account as a factor in determining contact and residence issues.

Such a test would in my view provide a charter for the abuse of children and particularly the very young. While I took a slightly more restrictive view than that taken by the High Court in M *and* M, it is obvious that a court exercising family jurisdiction bears a heavy responsibility to protect children. In many cases, the age of the child and the circumstances alleged make it impossible for the court to make a definite finding that abuse has occurred. It is for this reason that there are very few successful prosecutions of abusers of very young children. On the other hand, the court may be left with a very firm view that it would be unsafe to leave the child in the care of the alleged abuser. In my view it would be unthinkable to do so in such circumstances. The detrimental effects of child sexual abuse on children are well documented and no child should be left at risk of being subjected to this treatment.

Hirst is correct in his assertion that the Court's task in this area is rendered more difficult by the unsatisfactory nature of the investigations carried out by state and territory child welfare departments in relation to children who are the subject of family law proceedings. In effect it has been the approach of such departments to abandon the investigation to the Family Court, usually because of insufficient funding. At the same time the Court does not have an investigative arm. This is an unsatisfactory situation for both children and those accused of abusing them.

However it is also fair to say that the Court has been active in its attempts to overcome this problem, as the Magellan Project indicates. Its success has been very dependent upon the Court receiving the co-operation of the respective state and territory departments, which in the case of Victoria was forthcoming and very much contributed to the success of the project. Incidentally, like most of Hirst's work, his account of the naming of the Magellan Project is mythical.

As Hirst points out, the Family Law Council has proposed the setting up of a federal agency to investigate these allegations. I should have thought that a better solution would be for the federal government to properly fund the relevant state and territory departments to carry out these functions.

In my view, however, contrary to the view expressed by Hirst, these difficulties have led the court to adopt what some might regard as an overly restrictive approach to child sexual abuse allegations, as is evidenced by the decisions of the Full Court of the Family Court in N and S and the Separate Representative (1996) FLC 92-655, Re W (2004) FLC 93-192 (which was an appeal from one of my own decisions at first instance) and V and V (unreported delivered 25 November 2004). These decisions suggest that the Court has (probably impermissibly) adopted a much more restrictive approach than that prescribed by the High Court in M and M.

I consider that far from making biased decisions against fathers accused of abuse, a case could be made that the Family Court has not been protective enough of children in these cases.

It is nonsense to suggest, as Hirst does, that the mere making of an allegation of sexual abuse leads to an assumption by the Court that it is correct. It is true that the Court Rules prescribe that where such an allegation is made that notice of it be given to the Court and to the other party. This is no more than the provision of procedural fairness and also enables the Court to discharge the mandatory statutory requirement on it to notify relevant state and territory departments of allegations of child abuse.

However, beyond this the Court takes no action on such allegations unless an application is made supported by evidence on oath to restrict or end contact. When that happens and the allegations are serious, the Court has little choice but to either suspend contact or provide that it be strictly supervised until the allegations can be properly tested. To do otherwise would be to place the children in question at serious risk.

It is here that the Magellan Project has proved its worth, for it involves the case being promptly referred to a judge who will co-ordinate appropriate investigations by the state or territory department or other experts and ensure that the allegations are dealt with speedily. It was found that this led to much earlier determination of these cases and fewer of them going to court. When they do go to trial, the allegations are fully tested.

At trial, the judge is of course bound to apply the principles set out by the High Court in M *and* M as further expounded by the Full Court in subsequent cases. If a change in the law is considered appropriate, the Australian Parliament has had every opportunity to make it since 1988 and has not done so.

However, I think that there are grave dangers to children in making the test more restrictive as Hirst urges.

In conclusion, I consider that Hirst does a grave disservice to Australians and particularly to Australian women and children. The attacks made are emotional, far from child-focused and contain a surprising degree of misogyny. It is more than time that the family law debate was returned to objective ground where arguments are based upon evidence rather than myth.

One would expect, at least, that any critique purporting to be *academically* founded, like Hirst's, should emanate from someone whose research track record has at least touched upon the topic of family law in the past.

Alastair Nicholson

Bettina Arndt

"There's no doubt injustice has been done to men. The classic situation is the good father who sees his children every day and then Bang! The couple separates, the court gives him every second weekend. To have a dear little child that you love and suddenly your contact to him is so restricted. It's a basic cause for the anger so many men feel about the Family Court."

The speaker is not one of the disgruntled litigants so blithely dismissed by our former chief justice, Alastair Nicholson. This is retiring Family Court judge Geoffrey Walsh, who wrote to me nine years ago, contemplating the mistaken direction taken by his court. He summed up the error as follows – "the woman has had all the power, the man almost none." A mother with custody, he explained, was allowed to regulate access, live anywhere she liked, make decisions about day-to-day living and get a greater slice of the matrimonial cake. "More often than not that power is exercised unreasonably," he observed.

In the past nine years little has changed. The injustice continues. It is good to have our complacency about this appalling state of affair shaken by John Hirst's indignation. As an outsider, he investigates the Court and is blown away by discovering example after example of breathtaking disregard of men's basic rights. He finds a court where vile accusations are made against men with impunity, where perjury has no consequences. A court where men have to pay and pay to try persuade the Court to enforce its own orders. A court which even allows a woman to rename her child if it suits her.

He rightly thunders over the sheer stupidity of a system that allows lawyers to score points by fighting over where children will live. "Settling disputes between parents over the care of children in an adversarial way is madness." It is good to be reminded of the lunacy of it all.

But the solutions aren't so easy. I have long been a vocal supporter of a rebuttable presumption of joint custody. But the argument that gives me pause is the risk that this could lead to more litigation – that even more couples would end up in court if joint custody was the starting point. Any solution that prompts even more couples to fight in court over their children has to be avoided.

A very strong argument can be made that more parents will end up sharing parenting more equitably after divorce if they can be forced to listen to their own children, or taught to understand their needs. All the research shows very clearly that most children express a clear desire to be with both parents – which does not necessarily mean split time but flexible arrangements built around the children's needs rather than parental desires. When children's views are properly heard, many parents do approach things more sensibly. That's the essence of the approach the government is now backing, with the network of sixty-five new Family Relationship Centres, aimed at helping parents work out arrangements that are in their children's interests. These centres would be based around child-focused mediation devoted to determining what children need in terms of care, which is very different from the classic mediation that involves a negotiator simply helping battle out agreements.

Hirst is wrong to dismiss this as nothing new. The proposed mediation is different from what used to be offered by the Family Court, which was rarely child-focused and often distinctly biased against men. The approach being proposed is one that has already been shown to be effective, even with some of the most difficult cases that have spent years in and out of court. Apart from the child-focused mediation, high-conflict parents would be referred to a child-inclusive program, involving experts working intensively with the entire family, which is custom-made for the more troubled families that presently end up in court.

We know this works. For some years now, the Family Court has been referring some of their most difficult cases to such programs and finding parents do actually shift ground. We're not usually talking about huge changes but certainly less of a war zone, with parents far from friends but at least capable of reaching some arrangement with each other. And what's just as important, the mediation provides somewhere parents can go back to if arrangements become unstuck and they need further help. There's solid American research showing good quality mediation does result in fathers having more active and flexible long-term involvement in their children's lives, a far better result than was achieved through court battles.

But Hirst is quite right in warning that people should not be allowed to use allegations of violence or abuse to avoid this more civilised and effective approach. While it is often claimed this mediation is inappropriate in cases where there has been violence, the centres like Unifam which have been using child-centred mediation with cases referred from the Court are well used to handling people where AVOs have been issued, often on both sides, and still achieve successful outcomes. What is needed in these cases is that after proper investigation the Family Court should determine whether the abuse or violence actually took place, impose real penalties where there have been false allegations, and then refer such cases back to these special mediation programs. Court orders do nothing to help these troubled families find a way to parent effectively after divorce – but these programs can help, even when violence or abuse has occurred.

It was also pleasing to see Hirst shoot holes in so-called research claiming only 9 per cent of allegations of abuse were false. The issue of false allegations regarding abuse and violence has received attention from numerous inquiries into the Court, all of which have concluded this is a very real problem. A woman claiming abuse or violence often gains a significant advantage in denying her partner contact with the children. It is most unfortunate there has been no response to recommendations made to dealing with this very serious issue which brings the Court into such disrepute.

But Hirst struggles in dealing with the complexities of the child-support system. He mentions that men on low incomes cannot afford to live decently and make a substantial contribution to his former household. "Either the government has to discourage divorce or bear more of its costs," he suggests.

Well, the government is certainly working on discouraging divorce, which is why the new relationship centres are planned to include all sorts of counselling and referral services to try to shore up shaky marriages. And the government is already paying mightily for the costs of divorce. A staggering 40 per cent of payers are liable for only a token $5.00 a week payment due to their low incomes. According to the 2003 parliamentary committee report, *Every Picture Tells a Story*, the annual cost to the government of supporting separated families is over $2.7 billion a year. Most of the low-income families simply can't afford the costs of running two households and it is the government which is paying the bill.

At present a government committee is in the process of investigating the current child-support formula, aiming to recommend changes based on the actual costs of children, and taking into account factors such as the costs of contact which were not properly acknowledged in the previous formula. The recommendations from that technical committee, which comprises most of the key players with expertise in the area, will address some of the glaring faults in the current system. For instance, currently there is a reduction in child support when children spend more than 109 nights with the contact parent. This creates a cliff effect with fathers being restricted to fortnightly access so mothers won't lose money. Breaking this nexus is critical to encouraging more shared parenting.

John Hirst is right to applaud some of the changes taking place in the Family Court — notably the new inquisitorial approach currently being piloted. And the new Chief Justice certainly is a breath of fresh air. But there have always been some judges free of the anti-male bias that afflicts many of their colleagues, judges who do play it straight down the line. Some show real determination to shake up the Court's appalling record on enforcement of contact orders by imposing real penalties for breaches — a very welcome change. Yet this still means a visit to Court is a lottery, with men rarely the winners. That's why other solutions must be found. Let's leave the Family Court to the kangaroos … and seek answers elsewhere.

Bettina Arndt

Joanna Fletcher & Allyson Foster

John Hirst introduces his *Quarterly Essay* by saying, "Until recently I knew only as much or as little about the Family Court as anyone who follows current affairs." This becomes more and more evident as one reads his essay rather offensively titled *"Kangaroo Court"*.

To correct all of Hirst's legal errors and misleading statements would make for dull reading. We will therefore restrict ourselves to just one matter: Hirst's implication that women *get it all* when they separate while men just get pursued by the "ruthless and relentless" Child Support Agency. On the contrary, many resident parents and their children live in poverty after separation, and inaction by the Child Support Agency compounds this problem.

Australian Institute of Family Studies research shows that women are more likely to suffer financial disadvantage after divorce than men. Department of Family and Community Services data shows that 74 per cent of people entitled to child support (91 per cent of whom are women) raise their children on incomes below $20,000, with the average payment of child support being just $57.23 per week, while the average cost of raising just one child on an average income was calculated by the National Centre for Social and Economic Modeling as being $183 per week.

Far from the Child Support Agency being "ruthless and relentless" in its pursuit of child-support payments from non-resident parents, 41 per cent of resident parents receive no child support. In 2001 some $670 million had not been collected or passed on to children and $74 million was written off, not to be collected.

Individual anecdotes can be powerful but we don't want to trade heart-rending stories (although we have many to tell) because we believe that public debate and law reform should be informed by proper research and empirical evidence.

Joanna Fletcher & Allyson Foster,
Women's Legal Service Victoria

Justin Dowd

The Family Court has been dogged by controversy from the time of its inception to the present day; it had a controversial birth and as it turns thirty in 2005, it remains the most contentious court in the country. This is not really surprising; established through the efforts initially of the late Lionel Murphy, himself a controversial figure, the Court touches the heart of the nation. It is the Court that "ordinary" people are most likely to end up in. (It is said that the distinction between the criminal courts and family courts is that in criminal courts one sees the worst people acting at their best, and in the family courts the best people acting at their worst.)

This is at the heart of the problem in the family law jurisdiction today. If it were possible to legislate that people should always behave reasonably, or with their children's (or former partner's) best interests at the forefront, there would be no need for the family law system at all.

But that doesn't happen and it is necessary for society to regulate the separation of couples, of families, when the people involved are least amenable to regulation. It can be overlooked in the debate about the "Family Court" that each of the parties comes to the system with his or her own background, broken dreams, new aspirations. It is enormously difficult to provide much satisfaction in any case; the best the system can do is to provide a decision.

John Hirst's essay *"Kangaroo Court"* makes many valid and poignant points about the lives of the people that are affected as they work themselves, or are worked, through the family law system. In truth, once a person becomes a litigant in the Family Court, there are only two ways out … reach an agreement or have a stranger impose a decision. It is true that "reaching an agreement" is often, in reality, giving up, for reasons of a feeling of hopelessness, spiralling costs and total loss of control.

It should be recognised that the Family Court of Australia was established as a specialist court, with facilities, resources and expertise in the area of family law.

At the time of its establishment and early development, and particularly during the time of the attorney-generalship of Lionel Bowen, the Court had extensive counselling facilities (one-half of its counselling was done with couples prior to any litigation), it had regular and frequent country circuits and it was staffed to a level that allowed a degree of continuity and expertise. Sadly, these conditions were eroded over time.

It should also be recognised that the Family Court, like the Federal Magistrates Court established in 2000, operates within the parameters of the *Family Law Act*. The Family Court is a statutory court, meaning that, unlike courts of common law or equity, it cannot embark on a general search for "truth" or even (sadly) "justice" but can only administer and interpret the law that has been provided by the legislature. *"Kangaroo Court"* misses or confuses that point occasionally. For example, it is not open to the Court to "enforce" its own orders in the sense that it could initiate some form of prosecution. There is no legislative mandate for that. Similarly, arguments about the reintroduction of "fault" as a concept must remain with the parliament, and not be used as stones to throw at the Court itself.

That said, it must be recognised that many litigants leaving the Family Court do so with a sense of not having been heard, of their own concerns and issues not having been relevant to the issues heard by the Court.

The Court (if it had one voice) would, I suspect, be proud that it espouses that the welfare of the child is paramount. As a society, we would also adopt that principle without question. But *"Kangaroo Court"* raises very valid questions about what this might involve. The Court HAS shown a reluctance to respond to complaints by non-resident parents about breaches of contact orders. It HAS regularly imposed meaningless sanctions on resident parents, even after *Family Law Act* reforms laid out a new and seemingly tougher emphasis on enforcement of parenting orders. It is true that the response of the Court is often, "What do you want me to do, send the mother to gaol?" or "If I fine her, should you pay more child support?" In truth, mostly, the fathers don't want those things either, they just want to see their kids regularly, without the need to be "allowed" to see their own children. There is no procedure to bring enforcement of contact cases quickly before the Court (to comply with the Court's rules means there is necessarily a delay of at least four weeks) and the procedure is document-heavy and therefore expensive. The penalties imposed are almost meaningless, almost all of the time. The suggestion that recognising "the welfare of the child" includes seriously supporting its own orders is a good one.

It is true, in my experience at least, that the Court does not react to perjury.

"Truth" is difficult in this area of law as the things that litigants are trying to prove have more to do with intentions and attitudes than with objective facts. In 2003 there was a case in which a mother accused the father of raping her during a contact change-over period. The father denied the allegation and there was much written and oral evidence from the mother about the allegations. However, the mother did not know that the father had a tape-recording of the whole incident that demonstrated beyond any doubt that the mother's allegations were fabricated. Notwithstanding this, the mother's application for residence orders was successful and the judge recommended no action in respect of the false allegations. (As a postscript, the father, through his solicitor, referred the documents to the Commonwealth Director of Public Prosecutions who also declined to take any action.)

The Court's easy acceptance of the frailties of its witnesses has led it to a position where there is not even a culture of truth, and therefore no concern when truth is absent.

The Child Support Agency, it is said, is the government instrumentality about which most complaints are made. There is a perception in many of its users, both payers and payees in my experience, that it is the "ruthless and relentless" organisation described by "*Kangaroo Court*". The Agency, like the Court, suffers from being the public face of the legislation that supports it. If the legislation is cumbersome, confusing and inflexible, then it is likely that the Child Support Agency will exhibit the same attributes.

One of the most debated issues surrounding child support and contact issues concerns the fact that the legislation makes it clear that the two issues are not to be related. That is, the liability to pay child support continues to exist even where contact is not occurring. This is a major grievance with many litigants, who feel keenly that this is an unjust result. However, it is for the parliament to fix, not the courts or the Child Support Agency. There is a deeper issue involved, though, and that is whether the payer's relationship with the child is supported, in the child's mind, by these payments. I also think that it may be deeply satisfying in the long term for a non-resident parent to be able to say, "I didn't let them take away my right to support my child" – although I acknowledge that this might be cold comfort in many cases.

Some judges, it should be said, have shown much mettle in recent years in preventing resident parents relocating when this would affect adversely the non-resident parent's relationship with their child. The Court has also been such a regular supporter of the desirability of a child's surname not being changed that those orders are now only rarely sought.

Improvements are always possible in the area of family law, and the need to re-consider where a child's best interests actually lie is one of the most critical of these. The Court's enforcement regime remains an unsolved problem at this time.

Justin Dowd

Liz Olle et al.

We feel compelled to respond to the inaccurate claims about violence and family law made by John Hirst in the most recent edition of *Quarterly Essay*. The evidence relating to the practice, procedures and outcomes of Family Court hearings is vastly divergent from Hirst's assertions and claims.

First, women and children do not routinely make up allegations about child abuse or domestic violence, and the court does not routinely deprive men of contact with their children without credible evidence. The vast majority of the allegations are heartfelt pleas for protection from genuine experiences of violence and abuse. Secondly, and of most concern to us, the myths that this essay perpetuates endanger women and children who are victims of domestic violence. These two points are supported by extensive contemporary research. This response explores just some of that research and evidence.

Given the levels of child abuse in the general community, one would expect a significant portion of Family Court cases to involve allegations of abuse, but in fact such allegations are relatively rare. The evidence from all four Australian studies on this issue shows that among those allegations actually raised in court, "false" allegations are rare and they are made by fathers and mothers at equal rates. Residence and contact disputes involving allegations of child abuse represent 5 to 7 per cent of all disputes in children's matters before the Family Court of Australia, according to a study of disputes in 1995–96. In another Western Australian study of all cases in 1993 where children's residence or parental contact were in dispute, only 1 to 2 per cent involved allegations of child abuse. Cases in which child abuse or domestic violence are alleged without foundation do occur. Hirst provides detailed anecdotes regarding individual cases fitting this bill, but he neglects the wider evidence that such cases are rare. Allegations of child abuse rarely result in the denial of parental contact.

It is simply false to claim, as Hirst does, that women routinely, arbitrarily and maliciously use allegations of violence to deny men contact with their children.

His claim that it is quite clear that women are keeping children away from their fathers is not, and cannot be, supported by evidence. No credible research in Australia or elsewhere has demonstrated anything of the sort. To the contrary, many women go to great lengths to encourage and maintain father–child contact, even when their own personal safety is at risk.

On all the available evidence, the Australian Family Court does not pander to the whims of women, to the deliberate or even unintended detriment of fathers. In fact the converse is more accurate. The inherent problems in demonstrating to a court's satisfaction that violence and abuse exist are legion. The standards of evidence employed by the Family Court deter mothers from raising the issue with their own lawyers, or in court. Women report being pressured into arrangements they don't believe provide for the safety of their children in order to satisfy the Court's need for "reasonableness". Even where the Court accepts that violence has occurred, it still may award contact between children and the father on the dangerous assumption that a violent father is better than no father at all.

The Family Court already makes decisions that compromise the "best interests of the child"; facilitation of contact is often given priority over safety concerns. The regressive changes to family law advocated by Hirst can only make this situation worse. The federal government's proposed family law reforms recommend that where allegations of abuse are not able to be substantiated, residency may be awarded to the other party and costs will go against the party raising the allegations. This will further deter women from speaking out about violence and deny them opportunities to protect their children.

The best interests of children must begin from a position of safety. Any right to contact must not override the right of a child to be safe from abuse, or from witnessing violence against their mother. When Jayson Dalton applied for interim custody of his two young children, Justice Jordan of the Family Court said, "You've told me that he's been violent to his wife, but you haven't really told me … He's been a hard father, OK, but he hasn't really been violent to his children. They stay with him until she is well." (Liz Jackson, "Losing the Children", *Four Corners*, August 2004). There were at least two domestic violence orders against Jayson. Within two months he had killed his children.

Hirst's assertion that it is non-biological fathers who are violent or abusive to children is incorrect. Research, nationally and internationally, consistently identifies the biological father as the most likely offender in intra-familial sexual abuse. There have been many other child-murder cases, both in Australia and internationally, where children have been murdered by their (predominantly) biological fathers after a court failed to recognise the violence against their mothers as a relevant factor in determining contact arrangements. In many of the cases where the children were murdered, there was no violence directed at the children prior to separation or residency and contact negotiations, but substantial evidence of a history of violence used by their father against their mother.

While Hirst acknowledges that parents who have used violence towards children should be prevented from gaining "access" to them, he repeatedly discounts the rate, level and impact of violence within families. Ample research demonstrates that witnessing violence by one parent against another has lifelong impacts on children's health and wellbeing. Research also shows that the parenting style of fathers who use violence or abuse against their partners can be harmful, as these fathers tend to be more authoritarian, inconsistent and critical towards their children. There is no recognition of this in Hirst's discussion.

"*Kangaroo Court*" is not supported by evidence. It contributes to myths that already harm families; myths that gain credibility and durability by constant reiteration. The wide coverage of these assertions (nationwide press and radio coverage, etc.) means that Hirst's message will have reached into the homes of many of the women and children whose rights and safety he so blithely denigrates, contributing to a perception that the community does not take seriously the experience of violence and abuse.

Hirst minimises the effects and extent of violence, and advocates for retrograde and punitive procedures – for example that makers of 'malicious allegations' should be charged with perjury – which reflect precisely those behaviours – for example the threat of heavy-handedness – shown to exacerbate violence, abuse and relationship breakdown.

Furthermore, his essay reinforces a populist discourse broadcast by fathers' rights groups that denies the rights of children and women and feeds into irresponsible chatter about maligned fathers and myths about vindictive mothers. His claims are wrong: not supported by the evidence and based on anecdote rather than analysis.

Liz Olle, Allie Bailey, Mandy McKenzie and Margot Scott, Domestic Violence and Incest Resource Centre (Vic.); Dr Michael Flood, Australian Research Centre in Sex, Health and Society, La Trobe University; Dr S. Caroline Taylor, University of Ballarat, Research Fellow; Julia Tolmie, University of Auckland, Senior Lecturer in Law; Danny Blay, "No To Violence", the Male Family Violence Prevention Association, Manager; Marg D'Arcy, Centre against Sexual Assault, Royal Women's Hospital, Victoria, Program Manager

Barry Maley

Since the far-reaching changes to family law in 1975 and the creation of the Family Court, a body of evidence has accumulated of serious problems in the proceedings of the Court, declining marital conduct and the deteriorating status of marriage. The divorce rate has tripled, age at marriage has risen by an average of seven years for men and women, and fertility has halved within a generation. Almost one child in three today is separated from one of its natural parents – most often the father. Correlation is not proof of causal connection. But it is likely that the change in legal rules and administration is among the factors leading to the instability of marriage and retreat from it.

In an important sense, the problems with the Court that Hirst identifies are subsidiary to a more fundamental issue that is central to what is wrong with family law and the decline of marriage. It is the source of multiple injustices that include, but go beyond, those of custody arrangements and false charges of abuse of children. Towards the end of his essay, Hirst acknowledges this. He expresses concern about the "no-fault" principle governing divorce since 1975 and gives an illustration of some of its perverse consequences. To understand fully the implications and deficiencies of "no-fault", we need to think again about what marriage means and what is required to ensure justice in divorce.

An application for divorce used to require proof of serious misconduct ("fault" – such as adultery, desertion, habitual intoxication, abuse, etc.) in a marriage before the divorce could be allowed. The reason for this requirement was that serious misconduct in a marriage went to the heart of what marriage was about. It was a breach of the good faith and "cherishing" so important to the expectations of the parties to a marriage. But marital misconduct disappeared completely as a legal category in divorce in 1975 and henceforth all that was required for divorce was "irretrievable breakdown" demonstrated by one year's separation of the spouses. Needless to say, serious misconduct did not disappear as a reality in many marriages; nor as a burning issue in the minds of its casualties, albeit one that could no longer be raised in divorce proceedings and settlements.

Family law is the business of the federal parliament, and marriage and family life are nothing if not rule-governed institutions under law. As common sense would suggest, and as Hirst has shown in his examples, if the rules governing marriage are inadequate or poorly formed, or if sound rules are not enforced, marital conduct and family life will be adversely affected. The purpose of social rules, both informal and legal, is to shape conduct in conformity with accepted moral principles. In most societies, marriage, with its "vows" and rules governing marital conduct, serves (or used to serve) two fundamental objectives of social importance and individual value. They are: to confer benefit to the spouses by promoting life-long heterosexual companionship, mutual good faith and mutual care between wife and husband; and to protect the welfare of any children through the enduring partnership of their biological parents.

Given these objectives, breach of the rules of conduct in marriage should not be irrelevant to a court considering an application for divorce. If this is not the case, and it becomes the rule that serious misconduct within marriage will be of no account to the terms of ending a marriage, conduct during the marriage is less likely to fulfil the compact that is the purpose of the marriage. This will steadily destroy the status of marriage as a special, rule-protected, life-long commitment, and imperil the welfare of the partners and their children. It will come to be seen (and, indeed, is now seen) as an enterprise full of hazards and disappointments – some of which Hirst has revealed. Conversely, if the law takes notice of serious misconduct by signalling to potential perpetrators that they may be required to mitigate the damage done to the legitimate marital expectations of their spouses, an incentive is created for better conduct and better marriages.

The law, in short, can be an educative and morality-upholding force, no less in the compact of marriage than in other civil and commercial relationships intended to achieve mutually beneficial ends. In such formal contracts, a breaching party is expected by the law to limit as far as possible the damaging consequences to the other party whose way of life and fortune may depend upon performance of the contract. This should be no less the case in marriage, which is, for the great majority of women and men, the most important compact and the most serious investment they will ever make. If it comes to dissolution, the case for just treatment of the parties is unanswerable.

Unlike other "contracts", a marriage can be unilaterally and opportunistically ended at will by one party simply leaving the family home for a year and applying for a divorce that cannot be refused. The winding-up of the marriage and the settlement will be completely uninfluenced by the conduct of the party who has unilaterally "breached" unless the behaviour is shown to be relevant to the question of custody and "the best interests" of the children. Otherwise, marital conduct cannot be an issue. In short, faithful and conscientious investment in a marriage and the legitimate expectations of a spouse can be destroyed unilaterally and family law will take no notice of the damage inflicted – not even a finding that the spouse has been ill-used. Serious misconduct is a common marital reality but legally irrelevant and without legal consequence.

To suggest that serious misconduct should be relevant does not mean that we should return to the pre-1975 situation where fault had to be proved in order to get a divorce. It is possible to fashion legal and just remedies for the two critical problems of no-fault divorce – the failure to acknowledge the reality and consequences of serious marital misconduct; and unilateralism – while retaining the essentials of the present system of divorce after one year's separation.

The issue of opportunistic unilateralism could be overcome by requiring that formal divorce proceedings after one year's separation must begin with a *consensual* application by the parties and include agreed terms of settlement. But if consensus fails to be achieved, an application can be made by only one party on the understanding that this will trigger a Court inquiry into the reasons for absence of consensus and the breakdown of the marriage. In either case, whatever the finding if a Court inquiry is involved, the outcome would be divorce after the usual one-year separation. It may be that, as a result of the Court inquiry following a single, non-consensual application, a settlement will be ordered mitigating the losses of a spouse who has been shown to have suffered damage as a result of the serious misconduct of the other spouse. Conversely, the Court may find that serious misconduct is not an issue and allow the divorce to proceed on the basis of the application by only one party; with either a consensual settlement if that is possible or, failing that, one ordered by the Court.

The purpose in retaining recourse to a single, non-consensual application is twofold: to safeguard exit from a failed marriage by either spouse if a consensual settlement is impossible; and to provide an opportunity for a claim of serious misconduct to be aired and judged. Submitting a single application triggering a Court inquiry would therefore be a serious step. If submitted for mischievous or deceitful motives, or if false claims were made, a penalty might be incurred.

The obligation to forge a consensual divorce will take place in the shadow of a possible Court inquiry if agreement is not achieved. This creates a strong incentive for a couple in trouble, or an unhappy spouse, or perhaps an otherwise opportunistic and selfish spouse, to search for a settlement that will meet the wishes of both parties. This means that each spouse, before an application is submitted, will be forced seriously to confront the costs and benefits of staying together against the costs and benefits of divorcing, and for each to better appreciate the effects of divorce upon the other, and any children. If one spouse is more keen than the other to get out of the marriage, he or she will have an incentive to offer terms of settlement attractive to the other spouse which the offering spouse is nevertheless willing to bear in order to divorce. In other words, neither spouse is subject to the will or whim of the other. Each is in a position of formal equality with the other to bargain for an outcome acceptable to both; and the outcome would be either a decision to stay together, or forge a consensual application, or submit a single application triggering an inquiry. If children are involved, questions of custody would be part of the bargaining about the settlement and here, too, an outcome acceptable to both would be much more likely. Such a situation mimics what happens every day in negotiations to end a troubled or breached commercial contract. The parties can reach a mutually acceptable, and therefore just, adjustment, or appeal to the Court to deliver justice and possibly mitigation to the party demonstrated to be most damaged by the breach.

These ideas have been misunderstood by some as "re-introducing fault-based divorce", which of course it is not. For the great majority of divorces, fault would not arise as a legal issue. Perhaps more than now, divorce would be by mutual agreement, thus implying a fair break, and with the bonus that we could be more confident that a party has not been unwillingly and unilaterally deserted without a say, or intimidated by a stronger partner. Divorce after one year's separation would still apply. Even if fault has in fact occurred, this system would give an aggrieved party the opportunity of pursuing mollification by negotiation with his or her spouse without it being raised as a Court issue.

In the pre-1975 divorce regime, only a fraction (about 10 per cent) of divorces were contested in Court under a system which (unlike what I am proposing) required that fault must either be admitted to the Court or proved by Court contest before a divorce would be approved. In what is proposed here, where proof of fault is not a necessary condition of getting a divorce, the fraction of divorces in which a fault claim might be raised would likely be miniscule. The mere presence of the opportunity is what matters, even if it is rarely used.

At the end of his essay John Hirst says: "I cannot see the way by which the Court can be rescued. Until there is fundamental change, it will continue to give offence. The Family Court is a monstrosity, a court of law that cannot by its no-fault charter be a court of justice."

What is proposed here would be complementary to, and extend, Hirst's proposed reforms. It would take the cause of matrimonial justice a step further towards empowering both spouses and confronting the fatal illusion of "no fault". It opens up a path to fairer negotiation between spouses about ending, after the present one-year separation, a marriage that is no longer tolerable to one or both. In the process of negotiating an agreed settlement, everything is on the table. In the background, supporting good faith and fairness in bargaining a way out of a marriage, is the ultimate protection of a right to petition a Court inquiry. Where serious misconduct, or "fault", is a real and vital issue to one or both parties, there is an avenue for bringing it before a court of justice and seeking from it a just finding and resolution. With mutual empowerment and negotiation, and a court required to judge serious misconduct if necessary, we would have all the ingredients for finding the best way out of failed marriages. Children would be beneficiaries and spouses would feel that their concerns have been acknowledged and dealt with as fairly as possible. We should expect, and demand, no less than this. Until we get it, marriage and family life will continue to decline and all will suffer, one way or another, from its disarray.

Barry Maley

Diana Bryant

Despite the length of John Hirst's essay, my response will be brief but not because
I accept the author's criticisms as valid. I do not.

I will make no comment on the many invectives in the essay as I am sure they
will be understood by readers as a headline-grabbing device, rather than a con
tribution to the substance of his arguments.

I intend to treat the author's criticisms of the Court as falling into three dis-
tinct categories although the author himself does not always make appropriate
distinctions.

First, the writer criticises many aspects of the current law including High
Court decisions the Court must apply. For example, he questions whether the
"best interests of the child" principle in the *Family Law Act* should be modified in
some categories of cases; if the "unacceptable risk" test is appropriate; whether
it is fair that the government provides a mechanism for payment of child support to be enforced while contact enforcement is left to the individual; if the
current penalties in the Act for contravening orders are sufficiently strong; and
even whether fault should be reintroduced in some form.

These are all matters for which there may be different views held by members of the community, or even individual judges, but it would be totally
inappropriate for the Court to express a view in a public forum about legislation
and decisions of a superior court which it is bound by law to apply in individual cases.

Secondly, the author criticises independent academic family law research.
Although there are many issues I have with the argument he makes, I do not see
it as the Court's role to defend attacks on research published by independent aca-
demics.

Thirdly, based on several stories of individuals whose versions of events he
accepts as complete and accurate, the author expresses opinions as to how the
Court operates unfairly.

In my view, just as it is inappropriate for a court to express views about the law it is bound to apply, it is equally inappropriate for a court through its representative to engage in a public debate with anyone who expresses a personal opinion, whether or not that opinion is expressed in a forum such as *Quarterly Essay* or simply in a letter to the daily newspaper or some other media outlet.

The role of courts, and the Family Court of Australia is no exception, is to hear and determine cases that people bring before it. Most importantly that means hearing evidence and submissions from both sides – not just one – assessing all of the evidence from the parties, lay witnesses and expert witnesses, making findings of fact when necessary where facts are in dispute and deciding the case according to law.

In the case of the Family Court, such decisions must be consistent with the provisions of the *Family Law Act* and any relevant Full Court or High Court authority, which would be binding on the trial judge. Finally a judge is required to deliver a judgment explaining why certain findings of fact have been made and why the ultimate decision was reached.

The difficulties and complexities of making a decision in an individual case, for example the need to protect children from harm where allegations have been made against a parent versus the continuation of an existing regime of contact, will be understood by reading the judgment. Indeed it is by reading judgments that the difficult issues judges have to decide and how they go about decision-making can be best appreciated.

I invite those who have read John Hirst's essay and who wish to know how the Court does explain its decisions, to inform themselves by reading the judgments on the internet or, as the Court is open to members of the public, by coming and listening to how cases are presented.

Diana Bryant

John Hirst

In my study of the Family Court I thought it important to characterise as best I could the mind-set of the judges. To guide me I had the numerous public speeches of Alastair Nicholson, the former chief justice, my sampling of the judgments given from the bench, and the various official reports that had examined the Court's proceedings, to which the judges had sometimes given evidence.

From the fathers' groups I heard accusations that the Court was a feminist conspiracy and that the judges were heartless monsters. These views I did not accept, though I could understand how they had been developed. My conclusions were that the judges were soft-headed about enforcing the Court's authority, that they operated with a narrow view of the child's best interests, which they assumed could be sharply distinguished from that of their parents, and that they protected themselves from criticism by claiming that they were caring for children and their critics were doing something else.

The responses of former judges Evatt and Chisholm to my essay can be taken as confirmation of this analysis on all points. I am finally dismissed as *adult-centred!*

The judges acknowledge the problem of enforcing the Court's orders but claim that given the difficulties the Court faces it cannot do any better. They dispute my report that the Court, even when considering penalties for disobedience of its orders, treats the interest of the child in the case as paramount. They quote the *Family Law Act* at me. There has always been in the legislation sufficient power for the Court to enforce its orders. It was a decision of the Court to make the child's interest paramount. My authority on the Court's approach to penalties was the enquiry conducted by the Australian Law Reform Commission, which reported in 1995 that judges and registrars considered "the paramount concern has to be the interests of the child in the particular case" (*For the sake of the kids*, p. 96).

But let us accept, as the judges claim, that when orders are breached they do balance the needs for enforcement against the interests of the child. Whether the Court gets this right, they suggest, could only be determined by examining each case. This is not the appropriate test. The tests are whether the Court's orders are generally obeyed and whether the authority of the Court is widely accepted. The answer is NO, NO. The approach of the judges confirms my view that the Court has no understanding of the need to maintain the integrity of the system which it operates. My position is not that the interests of the child should be of no concern in enforcement, but that they should not be the paramount concern.

The judges think that that I am being sensationalist in claiming that the orders of the Court are a joke. But I am only relaying the common talk which was reported by the Family Law Council in 1998 in these terms: "There is 'a fairly widely held view in the community that the Family Court is reluctant to enforce its own orders'." A joke seems a mild characterisation of the Court's operations as revealed in my story of Julian Aston. The child's mother took the child from Adelaide to the Northern Territory in defiance of the Court. When ordered to return she refused. When after many years she was asked to return so that the child could be assessed she refused. She actually said she would come if the Court paid for travel, accommodation and a lawyer. The judge muttered that the mother knew very well that the Court did not provide money to litigants. But the judge refused to make her come. Then in her judgment the judge regretted that she had to make a decision in the absence of the child!

The Court, as a child of the 1970s, reminds me of those schoolteachers who thought that if they were caring and understanding they would have no need to resort to disciplining their charges. If you ask one of those teachers why their classrooms are chaotic, they will tell you that the children come from disturbed families and that what they have to learn is not relevant, etc. But if you wait until the next lesson with a different teacher, you might well find the classroom becomes perfectly orderly and that with no overt signs of control the children are cheerfully doing their work. The Court has yet to try how its troubled and angry clients would react to true authority. It is the absence of authority that makes them seem ungovernable. I have the support of Justin Dowd on this. Wild accusations fly around the court because, as he reports, the judges have abandoned any attempt to encourage the telling of the truth.

The two judges claim to have difficulty in establishing my recommendations for enforcement. They rightly say I am not endorsing sharp punitive methods. They skip over my report of the course recommended by various public enquiries: "They wanted the Court to use a range of remedies, but still keeping fines and imprisonment as a last resort. Above all they pleaded with the Court to take enforcement seriously; to be firm and consistent." It is worth repeating that my criticism of the Court over enforcement simply echoes the conclusions of numerous enquiries. The two judges have more than me to answer. Broadly I support what these enquiries have urged. My own formulation, made clear elsewhere in the essay, is that the Court should be both robust and deft.

The present government considers that the Court can do better. In cases where a custodial parent is denying access to a child, the government plans to give the Court power to transfer custody to the other parent – but with the proviso that the best interests of the child must be paramount. I suggested that this would render the plan nugatory because the Court would say that the best interests of the child determined the child's present placement and that a move would damage the child. I suggested that where the Court had been persistently defied, the custody could be transferred to the other parent *so long as the other parent was adequate to the task*. The judges criticise my plan for not taking account of the child's wishes and feelings and for being *adult-centred*. But I go on to say

> If [judges] are intelligent and caring, they will choose carefully the cases on which they make a stand so that children are not damaged. Not many cases would have to be resolved in this way before custodial parents took an entirely different attitude to access than they do now.

That is, I was caring for the particular child and my purpose was to benefit the thousands of children and their fathers who currently don't see each other because access is denied. So my *adult-centred* approach would benefit far more children than their child-centred approach.

Why did the judges omit to mention this passage? It would not be because they deliberately wanted to misrepresent my position. I think it is because they truly do not see a problem in the Court's present practice and so they are not interested in any solution. In other courts soft-headed and hard-headed judges labour on particular cases without having to worry about the authority of their Court, which is institutionally secure. Only rarely will anyone defy other courts. The Family Court has a particular problem: it has to regain authority. So much evil and heartache flows from its absence. These will continue if the judges maintain the approach of Evatt and Chisholm.

While these judges were penning their reply to my essay, a father – one of scores – contacted me with his problem. He has access to his boy every second weekend with the pick-up point being the boy's school. But on Fridays the mother keeps the boy from school. The father knows where the mother and boy live, but he has been advised that his case would be damaged if he went to an unauthorised pick-up point. His question to me was should he spend tens of thousands on a lawyer to run a case to enforce the access orders that the Court has given him. Of course I was reluctant to give advice, but when pressed I inclined to the view that he would be wasting his money – which was his own fear. I should start sending these queries to former judges Evatt and Chisholm. Then perhaps they would see the damage that soft-headedness causes.

In my essay I urged the Court to consider child and parents together, each with their interests and needs. I was moved by the plight of fathers kept from their children, but in urging their case I was also advancing the interests of their children. As the pavement graffiti at my local shopping centre avers: FATHER EXCLUSION IS CHILD ABUSE. The judges remain confident that the interests of children can be determined apart from that of their parents. Their reply confirms my assessment that the Court considers parents merely as candidates for involvement in the child's life. The Court will consider the child first and expects the parents will still be good for the child no matter what the Court does to them. A dad may be sent broke by paying legal fees spent in order to see his child or he might find seeing the children only every second weekend heart-wrenching or he may be unhinged by the Court allowing false accusations to run against him, but none of this damage is relevant to the best interests of the child!

The judges hold to the view that parents have no rights – that is, as soon as separation occurs both parents lose even a presumptive right to see their children. They accuse me of advocating courses that would be in breach of the UN Convention on the Rights of the Child. However, that document does speak of the rights of parents. Article 5 states:

> States Parties shall respect the responsibilities, rights and duties of parents ... to provide, in a manner consistent with the evolving capacities of the child, appropriate direction and guidance in the exercise by the child of the rights recognized in the present Convention.

The rights of parents are not defined other than in this Article, but at a minimum, to have any meaning, the right would have to extend to *seeing the child*. I think it is the Court that is in breach of the Convention.

The judges specifically ask me what I would do where a parent has been accused of child abuse and the evidence is ambiguous and the experts divided or uncertain. My answer is, as made clear in the essay, that I would allow the parent access to the child unless on the balance of probabilities the parent was proved to have been an abuser. Alastair Nicholson, the former chief justice of the Court, considers that this would give "a charter for the abuse of children". Yet this is the approach of the state family and children's courts. Nicholson seems to have retreated somewhat from his judgment in M and M where with great insight he said that once allegations of sexual abuse have been raised it is difficult to get rid of the lingering doubt that they may be true. Nicholson seems to imagine that only a hyper-vigilance by the Court stands in the way of a systematic sexual abuse by fathers of their own children. He plainly is not moved by the research that I report that fathers are the least likely abusers among the men known to the child. This finding is flatly denied by Olle at al. who claim that (unspecified) research demonstrates the opposite. My evidence was taken from Patrick Parkinson, "Family Law and Parent-Child Contact: Assessing the Risk of Sexual Abuse", *Melbourne University Law Review*, Vol. 23, 1999, and Thea Brown, "Fathers and Child Abuse Allegations", *Family Court Review*, Vol. 41, No. 3, July 2003.

The ex-judges and other respondents point out that some of the changes I recommend are beyond the power of the Court to effect. I knew this and indeed I do recommend that the law be changed so that parents can see their children unless the Court decides on good grounds that they will do them harm; and that parents accused of sexual abuse can be kept from their children only if they are found on the balance of probabilities to have abused the child. The judges speak of the Family Court being constrained by the High Court. It would be more accurate to say that the High Court has endorsed the approach of the Family Court, which invented the doctrines of no rights for parents and keeping parents from children without proof of offence.

Alastair Nicholson denies the Court's paternity of the no-rights-for-parents doctrine. He claims that it is the *Family Law Act* that has determined that "the right to contact is one of the child and not of the parent". It would be more accurate to say that the Act gives the child the right of contact and is silent on the rights of the parent. It is the Court that has decided that the best interests of the child can be interpreted to exclude a parent who has done no wrong from seeing the child. If this matter had been clearly settled by the Act, why would the textbooks still need to cite a Court judgment as definitive: *Brown v. Pedersen*? In that case the Court declared, "This Court has long laid to rest any notion that a parent has a right to access." Sounds like the Court making law to me.

Nicholson argues that the point is of little consequence because in nearly all cases access is granted. But the zealousness with which the doctrine is proclaimed and defended is significant. The doctrine frees the judges to do their dirtiest work: keeping parents from their children though no fault has been proved against them.

Nicholson rehearses again all the difficulties over the enforcement of the Court's orders. He is wrong to assume that my recommendation is 'the automatic enforcement of orders'. Of course the Court should use its discretion. But its aim must be a general obedience. The judges should establish a regime in which the people who come before them are disciplining themselves; they should hesitate to defy the Court or to tell lies. True authority does not depend on constant punishment.

Nicholson considers that I should not have strayed from history into his bailiwick and so given some academic plausibility to an account "riddled with factual inaccuracies". He and others can be assured that I did not abandon the constraints of my discipline and I made no statement unless I had firm evidence for it. Not all the evidence was supplied in the limited footnotes available in my essay. Where specific claims of inaccuracy have been made (these are surprisingly few given that my failings are said to be abundant) I am supplying my evidence in this reply. Nicholson gets specific in one place where he writes, "like most of Hirst's work, his account of the naming of the Magellan Project is mythical." I took my account from Thea Brown and the other social workers who wrote the official report on the project: *Resolving Family Violence to Children: The Evaluation of the Magellan Project*, Monash University, 2001.

I am accused by Olle et al of not taking violence against women seriously. I had no wish to hide it and I support the precautions that the Court has taken to minimise the risk of its occurring. Sadly this response supports my assessment that concerns over male violence can be a cover for opposition to any change. These respondents simply deny the existence of the problems my essay highlighted. I refer them to all the other respondents (including the former judges) who may differ with me over the extent of the problems and their solutions but do not deny their existence.

I am pleased that in many cases my analysis has been accepted and given further support by people whose acquaintance with the Court is longer than my own. I must acknowledge the sustained campaign of Bettina Arndt in defence of

fathers. It was her opinion pieces in the press that first alerted me to the short-
comings of the Court. I have not been able to tell her anything she did not know,
but she generously says that a newcomer can highlight the lunacy.

Bettina Arndt is optimistic about the new Family Relationship Centres. She
reports (what I have also been told) that good counsellors and mediators can
deal with violent people, so the government does not have to provide that the
violent cases must bypass the centres and go straight to court. This would be a
loophole too easily exploited. She rightly points to the importance of breaking
the nexus between amount of contact and child support. At present the custodial parent gets less child support when the child spends more than 109 nights
with the other parent. This is an inducement to limit contact. I hope the current
review of the system will address this problem. The government's plan,
announced in the 2005 Budget, to encourage single parents into the workforce
will, if successful, reduce the need for these families to get outside support,
whether from the government or the separated father of the children.

My endorsement of the proposal that fathers holding access orders to see their
children should not have to pay child support if access is refused received no
support from these respondents. The two judges repeated the usual arguments
against it, including the one that I hoped I had answered: that children losing
child support would have no means of support (they would of course be supported by the social security system). The judges showed no glimmer of
disturbance at the injustice of a father having to pay support for children whom
he is prevented from seeing. Dowd sees some advantage to fathers in maintaining their payments even though they can't see their children: it keeps a bond
with their children and is a sign to them that they have not been rejected, which
may be the basis for resumption of a relationship later. I know some fathers do
willingly maintain payments for these reasons. As is common in family law matters, everyone assumes that if there were penalties they would have to be applied
in all cases where there are currently breaches. Why not think that with the
threat of the withdrawal of child support custodial mothers might allow fathers
to see their children?

There was guarded support for the policy of a rebuttable presumption of joint
custody. The confusion over terminology continues to cloud debate. The two
judges claim that the Court already follows my recommendation that both parents be involved in the upbringing of the child. That may be the formal position
when it awards joint guardianship, but the Court certainly does not secure for
each parent the amount of contact with the child that would allow the involvement to be meaningful. Joint custody in this proposal for reform means equal

time or something approaching it with the child. The proposal is rebuttable and hence adjustable according to the best interests of the child, though its ruling assumption is that it is in the interests of children to have contact with their parents (unless they can be shown to be a danger to them). I advocated the policy as a good starting point for negotiations, which might in many cases end with a result not very different from the present, but with both parents having a voice in the settlement and its adjustment.

Bettina Arndt reports that she has long been an advocate of the policy. She does not take up my point that it is unlikely to be taken seriously in the new relationship centres unless the Act or the Court or both endorse it. Her doubt is that if it were law, the policy would lead to more litigation. I fear this less so long as the Court does move to an inquisitorial method with judges hearing cases more expeditiously and cheaply. This might be matched with the appointments of case-workers who would have oversight of settlements where there is conflict. At the moment parties record (often literally on tape and video) every infringement of their ex-partner in the hope that a huge pile of offences will win their case if it comes again to court before a judge who knows nothing of it. There would be less of this if parties could complain to a case-worker who had the power to approach the Court about penalties or changes to settlements. At every level we must recognise the standard adversarial methods of a civil court are totally inappropriate for this business.

In the essay I made only passing reference to the need to reduce our high divorce rate. I predicted that joint custody would reduce divorce since parents would know that they were not going to be able to marginalise or remove the other parent of their children. The objection to this might be that children would be damaged by being kept in households of severe conflict. But many marriages today are declared to be over by one party with the other unaware until that moment that there was anything wrong. There has been no overt conflict at all. These are the opportunistic separations of which Barry Maley speaks. As I said in the essay I am very respectful of his views and I am glad that this forum has given him another chance to air them. Only he has been prepared to reconsider seriously the no-fault basis of the existing law.

The former judges and the present Chief Justice describe my essay as polemic and invective. Certainly my prose is not as calm as theirs. I confess that I cannot remain calm when I learn that cases of child abuse can run for years in the Family Court and end only *when the child grows up and calls a halt*. It is the calmness of the judges that concerns me. Beyond the particularities of their argument with me, they seem to have no realisation of the extent of the social and human disaster over which they have presided. But I take some comfort from the restraint of the present Chief Justice's response. If she is not going to sail into controversy as readily as her predecessor, I hope she will listen and watch more closely. The Court has a wide field of action and much could be achieved by a chief justice setting a new direction.

John Hirst

Bettina Arndt is a social commentator, now writing for Australian Consolidated Press magazines (*The Bulletin* and *The Australian Women's Weekly*). She has written a great deal about the Family Court and has been a member of the Family Law Pathways Advisory Group and the Child Support Ministerial Reference Group.

Gail Bell was born in Sydney, educated in pharmacy and education at the University of Sydney, and has worked as a pharmacist, drug educator, chemistry teacher, literacy tutor and occasional journalist. Her first book, *The Poison Principle*, won the NSW Premier's Prize for Non-Fiction in 2002. Her second book, *SHOT: A Personal Response to Guns and Trauma*, was released to critical acclaim in November 2003 and short-listed for the Nita B. Kibble award.

Diana Bryant is the Chief Justice of the Family Court of Australia.

Richard Chisholm was a judge of the Family Court of Australia between 1993 and 2004, and is now an honorary professor of law at the University of Sydney and a part-time commissioner of the NSW Law Reform Commission. He has been engaged in law reform, teaching and research, primarily in the area of family and children's law, since the early 1970s.

Justin Dowd has had experience in family law since 1975. He is a former regional registrar of the Family Court of Australia and is now a partner in Watts McCray, the largest family law specialist firm in Australia. He is a regular presenter of seminars and papers on family law issues.

Elizabeth Evatt is a judge of the World Bank Administrative Tribunal and a commissioner of the International Commission of Jurists. She was chief judge of the Family Court of Australia from 1976 to 1988 and president of the Australian Law Reform Commission from 1988 to 1993.

John Hirst is Reader in History at La Trobe University and the author of several books, including *Convict Society and Its Enemies*, *The Sentimental Nation* and *Australia's Democracy*, as well as many commentaries for leading Australian newspapers and journals. He was a member of the Prime Minister's Republic Advisory Committee and the chair of the Commonwealth Civics Education Group. He is currently a member of the Film Australia Board and the Council of the National Museum.

Barry Maley is Senior Fellow at the Centre for Independent Studies in Sydney and was formerly a senior lecturer in Social and Behavioural Sciences for seventeen years at the University of New South Wales. His books include *Ethics and Ecosystems*, *Family and Marriage in Australia* and *Divorce Law and the Future of Marriage*.

Alastair Nicholson was chief justice of the Family Court of Australia from 1988 to 2004. He has been also a judge of the Supreme Court of Victoria and the Federal Court.

Peter Ryan was the director of Melbourne University Press from 1962 to 1989. He is the author of *Fear Drive My Feet* and, most recently, *Brief Lives*. For fifteen years he was secretary of the Board of Examiners of the Supreme Court of Victoria.